CFS Unravelled

GET WELL BY TREATING THE CAUSE
NOT JUST THE SYMPTOMS OF
CFS, FIBROMYALGIA, POTS
AND RELATED SYNDROMES

By Dan Neuffer

Foreword by Professor Kati Thieme PhD

Third Edition

Elednura
Publishing

CFS Unravelled

*This book is dedicated to my loving wife Lindsay,
who stood by my side and lifted my sights to new possibilities
that ignited hope when there seemed none.*

Disclaimer

The ideas, concepts, and opinions expressed in this book are intended to be used for educational and information purposes only. This book is not intended to replace your physician and is not a substitute for medical diagnosis, advice, or treatment. It is sold with the understanding that the author and publisher are not rendering medical advice of any kind. The author has a science/technology degree and is not a medical doctor or a naturopath and has no formal training in the biological sciences or health-related fields.

Please consult your doctors first, and check with them before you embark on any of the diet, exercise, or other programs and processes described in this book. It is recommended that all patients consult with their medical doctor before discontinuing any prescription medication or starting any medication or supplementation.

Please note that the illness described in this book is often categorised as different illnesses including Myalgic Encephalomyelitis (ME), Chronic Fatigue Syndrome (CFS), Systemic Exertion Intolerance Disease (SEID), Chronic Fatigue and Immune Dysfunction Syndrome (CFIDS), Post-viral Fatigue Syndrome and Fibromyalgia Syndrome (FMS). It also includes the conditions identified as Multiple Chemical Sensitivities (MCS), Electromagnetic Hypersensitivity (EHS) and Postural Orthostatic Tachycardia Syndrome (POTS). It is the author's view that these are different symptom expressions of the same illness as described in this book.

The explanation given in this book for the cause of this illness is the result of extensive research and analysis. However, it has not been universally agreed upon and hence must be described as hypothesis and not fact. Please note that this will not be reiterated in order to maintain clarity and flow of the text.

If you have not been formally diagnosed with the illness by a medical doctor, it is recommended that you do this first. Whilst specific diagnostic criteria exist for some expressions of this illness (eg. POTS, fibromyalgia), diagnosis is often made after eliminating other diseases. This process of elimination is important to ensure that you are not suffering from some other disease that should be treated by your doctor.

The author, publisher, and other people or organisations involved in the making of this book shall have neither liability nor responsibility to any person or entity for any liability or loss or damage arising caused directly or indirectly as a result of the use, application or interpretation of the material in this book. Please read this book only if you accept this and the other statements in this disclaimer.

Acknowledgement

CFS Unravelled was written by drawing on the scientific work of hundreds of researchers and medical professionals and their textbooks, scientific papers, and other publications. Towards the latter part of my research, I also found numerous works, some going back decades that agreed with large parts of this work and gave me the confidence to persist and take this work to completion.

However, I have found the work of Professor Joseph LeDoux of New York University and the pioneering work of Dr Hans Selye especially helpful.

This book could not have been completed without access to numerous medical libraries and the help of their friendly staff, without whom I may never have found the answers presented here. Thanks to all of you.

Thanks also to all those who reviewed my early drafts, both for your feedback and your encouragement.

A special thank you to my editor Nancy Meshkoff for helping to make this third edition more reader friendly and concise, I hope we have the opportunity to work together on many more projects.

I would also like to thank all the persons experiencing Chronic Fatigue Syndrome and Fibromyalgia Syndrome who I have met over the last few years. You have inspired me to forge ahead and complete this book. Every conversation with you has given me a sense of urgency.

Most of all I would like to thank my wonderful wife Lindsay. So often we forget about the effect on the loved ones of people afflicted with chronic illness. Not only did Lindsay support (and endure) me through all those difficult years, it was her continued faith that there were answers out there that allowed me to find them. It was her faith in my ability to write this book that has allowed me to share my research. I will forever be grateful.

Foreword

By Professor Kati Thieme PhD

I am a University medical researcher dedicated to researching CFS and Fibromyalgia, ANS dysfunction, and other chronic conditions. What makes CFS Unravelled unique is that it is a book that breaks through the noise of the huge range of symptoms and dysfunctions that people with this illness experience, and focusses you on the underlying dynamics that the medical research communities have wrestled with for many decades. Understanding this is key for you to regain your health!

The book is also powerful to help the reader move forward because it is written to empower the patient, the importance of which is often underestimated. An 83-year-old patient of mine said: "We have the duty to make ourselves feel well." She was in the hospital because of a severe rheumatic disease (LORA) and had survived the concentration camps at Auschwitz during World War II. Despite her experiences and severe illness, she termed her life as a "happy life." These words gave me a lasting impression about how important it is to empower someone with an illness that affects every area of their life.

After more than thirty years of working with hospitals, academics and pain clinics, I find it remarkable how often institutions disregard patient heterogeneity and don't know about the valuable information in this book. Sadly, many practitioners still feel that patients' symptoms are 'all in their head', even though clinical evidence, neuroscience advances, and brain imaging clearly prove that this illness, along with its symptoms of pain, fatigue, immune dysfunction and others, is real.

All too often, after a 5-minute interview, an opiate prescription is written with a request to come back in 2 weeks "to see if we need to adjust your meds". Little is more dispiriting than watching the medical system toil month after month only to produce unsatisfying and even harmful interventions and medication that will never heal you. On the other hand, few experiences are more gratifying than watching how this syndrome can be effectively treated and seeing patients become pain free again.

In this book CFS Unravelled, Dan Neuffer provides the vital connections between the large range of symptoms and dysfunctions of this syndrome. He can be proud to have put together many materials from divergent fields to give the reader a comprehensive perspective of this syndrome. He delivers the science about how the dysfunctions produce the symptoms in a way that the layperson can absorb and get their head around.

The fact that he himself experienced the syndrome clearly comes through to the reader, but perhaps the most important and valuable aspect of the book is the focus on recovering your health rather than just treating symptoms. His belief that the illness is real on the one hand and treatable on the other is one I wholeheartedly share.

What's really important to note is that a complex and dynamic illness doesn't simply respond to a pill or a single intervention. Two core messages of the book for recovery from this syndrome that strongly reflects my own clinical experience, are

> 1.) the need for a tailored approach that considers individual patient differences; and
>
> 2.) the need to address the underlying root problem.

Our research, supports the dysfunctions described in this book. We can measure specific brain patterns and other physiological evidence of a depreciated autonomic nervous system (ANS), which reflect disparate patient dysfunction and symptoms. Fortunately, recent advances in neuroscience show that these changes in the brain and periphery are plastic and can be reversed.

As an example, our research suggests that chronic pain is learned. With chronic pain, the brain has learned not to inhibit peripheral and other inputs, and is constantly or intermittently in a state of pain. Over many years, this brain pattern has developed and is maintained due to the dysfunctions experienced as well as other factors. This brain pattern (conditioning) has nothing to do with psychiatric disease or personality, and yet both physiological and mind strategies can be used to affect change in how the brain operates. In our lab, we combine ANS stimulation, through the baroreceptors, with behavioural therapy. Our SET (Systolic Extinction Training) approach is to trigger neuroplasticity by doing rather than just thinking about cognitive changes. The combination of a physical and psychological approach to affect changes in the nervous system is proving to be amazingly effective in a subset of patients, and has opened the door for further brain training programs to effect neurological changes. Patients can become pain free again.

As medical researchers, finding answers to complex questions is a vital part of what we do. But ultimately what matters most, is that our research translates into practical treatments and strategies that patients choose to adopt and benefit from. Both patient education and empowerment are key, which is why I feel CFS Unravelled is such an important book for anyone experiencing this syndrome.

There is light at the end of the tunnel. Although the approach to get through the tunnel is individual, neuroplasticity clearly exists, and YOU can find a path to health.

I wish you success in your endeavour to help yourself or a loved one with this syndrome. I can say - without reservation - that this book, and, more specifically, the information and methods that it espouses, can change your life for the better.

Kati Thieme, PhD
Professor of Neuroscience and Medical Psychology
University of Marburg
April 2017
"recipient of the 2008 International Award for Fibromyalgia Research"

Preface to
the Third Edition

How can you heal, when you don't know what's wrong? Does it even make sense to start a treatment for a dysfunction or symptom if you don't know what caused it?

Perhaps such treatments are OK if they have a lasting effect right away. However, when the symptoms and dysfunctions keep returning, then it makes more sense to discover the underlying cause and address that.

Needing to know the cause is what kick-started my journey out of seven years of terrible illness with ME/CFS/fibromyalgia. The frustration of endlessly treating symptoms and dysfunctions made me passionate about sharing my understanding and encouraging patients and physicians to focus first on understanding the factors driving this illness.

When I first published *CFS Unravelled*, the explanation was a result of my own research into physiology. It was my own theory, my conclusion as to the only thing that could explain all the dysfunctions and symptoms. It was really written as a hypothesis, as opposed to being filled with references and proof.

For many years now, medical researchers have observed this illness, but because of the many secondary dysfunctions, the huge range of symptoms, and the diversity of the patient population, the wider medical community is only now starting to come together as to its root cause. Inevitably, opinions vary; some still suggest that this syndrome is not a sickness at all, but rather a collection of separate conditions, or a mental condition such as depression or hypochondria (which couldn't be further from the truth).

Perhaps the biggest reason for this lack of consensus is that recovery is not produced by a simple cure, but rather from a tailored combination of approaches. What I hope you gain is a focus that goes beyond symptom treatment and focuses on normalising the root dysfunction I describe.

Since writing *CFS Unravelled*, I have worked passionately to share my understanding, to share hope by sharing others' recovery journeys and ultimately to support individuals to create their own recoveries. Along the way, my research has continued and my understanding about the process of recovery has continued to expand. However, whilst this third edition is more concise, to make it more readable, I have kept the initial approach of following my quest for answers. I believe it will closely align to yours.

Whilst you will learn how most of your symptoms are generated through the root and secondary dysfunctions, many symptoms are not covered. I get questions about such symptoms every week and have learned that many of us feel that because we don't understand exactly how these are generated, that we are different somehow or that something else is going on. Of course, we can experience more than one illness concurrently, so it is always important to be fully evaluated by your doctor, but I hope that you gain the confidence needed to take more focussed steps towards recovery after reading this book.

When you listen to stories of how others have recovered on my website or elsewhere, you will discover that many of your own symptoms or experiences are shared by others, even the more peculiar ones. You will realise that you may not have to treat every symptom for a full recovery, even if you have been sick for many years.

Most importantly, I hope that you will understand WHY they recovered, rather than just HOW they recovered, even if they themselves don't.

Note to Readers

If you have had this illness for some time, you may already have come across some of the information, concepts and ideas contained in this book. However, recovery usually requires a full understanding of both the dynamics of this syndrome and a multi-faceted treatment rather than a magic-bullet approach. This is true even when you treat the primary cause of the illness.

Hence we strongly urge you to read this book from front to back without skipping ahead.

If you are reading the electronic version of this book, you can download the diagrams in it if you register as a book owner at

cfsunravelled.com/bookowner

(this will also automatically subscribe you to receive email updates regarding new resources and you may unsubscribe at any time.)

Registering at the above address will also give you access to a list of further recovery resources that I am continually adding to.

Contents

Part One:
Introduction

CHAPTER 1

Naming Convention

"What's in a name? that which we call a rose By any other name would smell as sweet."

- William Shakespeare

Much contention surrounds the names given to this illness— not only about whether each is appropriate, but whether different names describe different illnesses altogether.

The names include Chronic Fatigue Syndrome (CFS), Myalgic Encephalomyelitis (ME), Fibromyalgia or Fibromyalgia Syndrome (FMS), Systemic Exertion Intolerance Disease (SEID), Postural Orthostatic Tachycardia Syndrome (POTS), Chronic Fatigue and Immune Dysfunction Syndrome (CFIDS), Multiple Chemical Sensitivity (MCS) or Electromagnetic Hypersensitivity (EHS) and sometimes other names are used for early expressions of the illness, such as Post-Viral Fatigue Syndrome (PVFS).

Other conditions such as Gulf War Syndrome (GWS) and Complex Regional Pain Syndrome (CRPS) or Reflex Sympathetic Dystrophy Syndrome (RSD) also likely fall into the same spectrum of illness, but include specific triggers and secondary dysfunctions that make them more uniquely identifiable (similarly to POTS and fibromyalgia where specific symptoms can be dominant).

I believe that none of these names are fitting, as most are based on symptoms and not on cause. I also believe that, despite their varied symptoms, these illnesses all share the same cause. Even if you disagree with me, I ask you to keep an open mind whilst you read this book and try to follow my reasoning.

For simplicity's sake, this book will refer to this illness primarily as Chronic Fatigue Syndrome (CFS). Please forgive me if this is not the name you believe to be correct. Also, instead of 'patient' or 'sufferer', I will use the term 'person experiencing Chronic Fatigue Syndrome' (PEC), since thinking of yourself as a sufferer is ultimately not helpful.

CHAPTER 2

Getting Started On The Right Foot

W hy is it that, at a time when all the answers are supposedly at our fingertips, we often cannot get straightforward answers about our health?

Why is it that, when the medical industry and list of medical research organisations are bigger than ever, an illness like CFS is still 'a mystery'?

I believe the answer involves three main factors:

1. The complexity of the illness.
2. The tendency for medical research to be highly specialised and focussed as opposed to looking at illness as a whole.
3. The years of unjust labels applied to people with CFS that have strained the relationship between patients and the medical community, making communication even more difficult.

Writing this book has been a challenge. Whilst health care professionals can benefit from it, my aim is to explain this illness to people experiencing CFS (PECs).

If you are a PEC, you may have very little medical knowledge, or you may have spent years reading and experimenting. The one thing you may have built up is scepticism. That's why I have gone into some detail to show how the dots are connected in my hypothesis. If you can't see how the illness works, you won't act on the conclusions. And if you don't act, you won't benefit from the knowledge. I hope I have struck the right balance between detail and clarity.

Over the years, I have heard PECs criticise the conclusions and treatments of researchers and practitioners from around the world. The problem is that many valid and important ideas represent only part of the puzzle of CFS. To get well, you must have the full picture and understand all the steps required for recovery.

At this point, I'm going to ask you to clarify what you believe about CFS. Write down your answers to the questions below. If you don't know the answer, write your best guess, or write, "I don't know."

1.   *What is the central cause of CFS?*

2.   *What are the main things you need to do to recover from CFS?*

3.   *Has doing these things led you to a full and permanent recovery?*

Since you're reading this book, I expect your answer to Question 3 to be "No." This does not mean that your beliefs are all wrong, but they are probably incomplete. Your answers are the start of a framework that you can fill in as you read this book.

Treating problems in isolation doesn't work. Neither does treating secondary problems alone. You must treat the root cause and address your own personal triggers of the cause.

You must also treat things in the right order. It's a bit like cleaning the house for an important dinner guest: If you vacuum before you wipe the crumbs off the table, you won't end up with a clean floor.

The mechanism of this illness is complex—complex because the human body is complex. Researchers, doctors, and PECs often get lost in the details and never see the big picture.

It is the big picture that *CFS Unravelled* is written to deliver - a big picture made of many individual puzzle pieces. I have sought to make the picture detailed enough for you to be confident that it is correct, so you can gain the confidence to start taking more focussed action to recover from this dreadful illness now.

CHAPTER 3

My Story

In 2002, my wife and I were blessed with the birth of our son. Unfortunately, my wife experienced complications and several times nearly lost her life. The experience left both of us shaken. My wife took some time to recover. I experienced post-traumatic stress and suffered from flashbacks, nightmares, and other sleep problems, as well as a terror of further medical mishaps. This is not the best state for a first-time father with a sick wife and a newborn baby to be in.

Several months later I collapsed at work with severe intestinal distress. Constipation had distended my bowel and, whilst the symptoms subsided, I was left with a spastic colon and pain in my lower abdomen for some time.

Over the next year, life somewhat returned to normal, as did my and my wife's health. In late 2003, I went through a period of very high stress due to work and other projects that I had taken on. I regularly worked twelve hour days and kept up an aggressive exercise regimen that made me lose about eight kilograms of fat in less than three months.

When news hit the office that the spouse of one of my colleagues had been struck down with chickenpox, I was very concerned because I had never had chickenpox. Not wanting to expose my wife and son to it, I got the first of two vaccination shots.

Five or six days later, I developed strange symptoms. At first, I had trouble keeping up with my colleagues during our leisurely lunchtime walk. A few days later, I struggled to keep up with my wife on a gentle walk whilst pushing our pram. After this, I deteriorated even further and experienced a variety of flu-like symptoms, with severe exhaustion unlike anything I had ever experienced before.

My doctor told me that my illness was due to a throat infection, even though I had no throat pain or discomfort. He explained that my throat was extremely red and inflamed and prescribed antibiotics. They had no effect except to cause a rash across my chest.

After months of sickness, I sought the opinion of another doctor. He was young and very diligent and kind. He examined me thoroughly and made a full analysis of my blood, checking for viruses and other potential problems.

I tested negative to everything except Epstein-Barr virus, for which I showed a past exposure. The doctor said I was most likely suffering from some other virus and that my symptoms should abate.

As the weeks progressed, my symptoms increased and decreased but did not disappear. Work was a struggle, and I repeatedly took time off. I stopped exercising. My life consisted of dragging myself to work, then coming home and crashing on the sofa. Nobody could tell me what was wrong. After a while, I realised that nobody appreciated the full extent of my symptoms.

My doctor took more blood tests, but my condition worsened. Within nine months, I could no longer work full-time.

During the next four years, I went from one doctor to the next in the desperate hope that someone could help me. I also saw alternative practitioners, such as naturopaths, who identified lots of problems and offered lots of treatments, but none of them really helped.

Whilst I had occasional periods of reasonable health, my overall condition was clearly worsening. I was now significantly unwell even when my symptoms weren't flaring up. I suffered with extreme fatigue, bouts of debilitating pain and fever, night sweats that soaked my bed, and unsettling neurological symptoms such as brain fog. Finally, I accepted that I had CFS. I had avoided this label, since nobody had an explanation or cure for this illness. In hindsight, I wished I hadn't been so stubborn and had accepted that I had CFS sooner.

By 2008, I had resigned myself to having a lifelong condition. I vowed to make the best of a bad situation and to live my life as well as I could. But a few months later, to my shock, my health deteriorated to a new low. I became bedridden and barely able to speak. My body was racked by inflammation and I spent my days curled up in severe pain. My energy crashed to unprecedented lows. Even forming a thought was nearly impossible. My nights were dominated by night sweats and twitching muscles.

This time was probably my low point, not just physically but also emotionally. Any parent can appreciate my deep desire to make the most of Christmas for my young children. But that year, as I lay on the sofa unable to speak, I realised that I couldn't even fake a smile for the kids or participate in any way. I was just part of the furniture.

Being too ill even to communicate was truly a frightening experience. My head, throat, and body aches eased off in January 2009, and I was again able to get out of bed and speak, but I realised that living with CFS as best I could was not an option. Yet what was my alternative?

I remember slumping at my computer desk one afternoon in January, still in my pyjamas. I was gazing out of the dark room at the blue sky through a crack in the curtains when these words popped into my head:

"Daniel, you work it out yourself."

Preposterous, I told myself. I was hardly going to find an answer that not even the medical community had found. Teams of doctors and researchers with years of specialized education had studied this illness. I wasn't even a doctor.

Then I thought of the movie *Lorenzo's Oil,* in which an ordinary couple succeeds in finding a cure for their son's illness. Could a layman like myself work out a seemingly impossible problem?

One part of me felt a sense of unstoppable determination (or perhaps desperation); the other was full of doubt at the seemingly ridiculous notion. So I gave myself a little pep talk: I reminded myself that I had graduated university as valedictorian with a degree in physics, topped my class in quantum mechanics, and solved Schrodinger's equation in three dimensions.

Surely I could work this out! How hard could it be?

Bravely, I announced to my wife my big, bold goal. I told her I would work out what causes this dreaded illness and would find a way to get well despite five years of being sick. She gave me her full confidence.

I tried to convince myself that I had the same level of confidence.

CHAPTER 4

Solving the Mystery

L et me say that, whilst the world of physics may seem complicated and mysterious, the human body is truly, incomprehensibly complex. Any suggestion that we fully understand it is wrong. We don't even fully understand the functions of a piece of broccoli, which contains hundreds of phytochemicals.

My first step was to browse the Internet more methodically. Although I'd done this before to some extent, I noticed that I was now finding information I had not previously seen—about the biochemistry of energy production, for example. I browsed through roughly a thousand scientific papers and studied about twenty in detail. Reading them was like reading a foreign language.

My next step was to look through books on CFS. After five or six of these, I realised that most contained the same information, but not the answers I was seeking. I didn't want to know what was not working in my body; I wanted to know *why* it was not working.

Using my scientific training, I tried to identify the logical sequence that caused CFS. But despite all my hard work, I couldn't form a clear picture. By now I'd read everything I could lay my hands on. I started to feel dejected.

Some months later, however, my research began to come together and I had formed a rough idea of the cause of CFS. And so I decided to implement a variety of strategies to move forward with my recovery.

Around this time, I found a holistic doctor who focused on treating

PECs. After so many years of illness, it was great to speak to someone who didn't look at me like I was making it all up. He helped me rebuild many aspects of my health and highlighted the importance of diet. The treatments involved a large number of tests and supplements, and they weren't cheap, but my digestive system started to heal and my health improved.

Later that year, I had recovered the majority of my health. Whilst I'd made mistakes and had some setbacks, I was like a different person. I wasn't exactly running off to the gym, and I wasn't confident that I wouldn't get worse again, but I had a much better Christmas.

Forming an explanation of the root cause and dynamics of CFS gave me focus. It's amazing how you can surf the internet for years and find nothing, but once you know what you're looking for, it's right there. I found much support for my developing hypothesis and I even noticed that others had come to similar conclusions.

It was encouraging to see that others shared large aspects of my ideas. But why hadn't these ideas been embraced by the medical community? Why did I have to work this out for myself?

I felt that one reason was that some of the key discoveries did not fully explain the dynamics of CFS. Whilst several had identified the primary cause, the lack of a wider view of the illness meant that their treatment programs were too one-sided, especially for PECs who had been sick for long periods of time. I had identified many points that I felt were critical for recovery and had formulated a treatment program that had worked for me, but I could not tie everything together to my satisfaction. I wanted to be absolutely certain that I wasn't missing an important piece of the puzzle, so that I would stay healthy.

By mid-2010, not only was I fully recovered, I had survived a test of extreme physical and psychological stress. I'd gone through excessive physical work and hours of severe mental stress, yet I didn't crash like I would have done in the past. I was exercising, working full time, and doing everything I wanted to do. I had a year of good health under my belt and was improving further by the day. So after about six and a half years, I could finally say that I no longer had CFS. It felt odd and somewhat surreal. Part of me felt that if I announced that I no longer had CFS, I would get struck down again so everyone could say, "Hah! I thought you said you were well!"

Not only was I fully recovered, I had formed a more complete picture of the pathogenesis and dynamics of CFS. I felt a high degree of confidence in it, not only because I had used it to recover, but because it explained so many of the 'unexplainable mysteries' of CFS. I now felt confident that my health would remain strong.

I looked at my notes and drawings and wondered what life might have been like if I'd had this information when I first got ill.

Interestingly enough, during all my years of being unwell I never met another PEC. Even after I admitted I had CFS, I had never gone to support groups because I felt that sitting around listening to other people complaining wasn't going to help me. This was a mistake. If I had accepted that I had CFS earlier and exposed myself to more information, I would have saved myself years of suffering.

Now, with my new understanding in place, I started to meet people with CFS everywhere. I met five in one month and many more after that. Perhaps it had something to do with no longer keeping my illness quiet, or perhaps it was coincidence, but it had a profound effect on me.

It gave me the opportunity to discuss my experience with others. It is profoundly comforting to know that you're not the only one going through something so upsetting and bewildering. Sure, I'd known that many people have CFS, but sharing my individual symptoms and talking to someone who *truly* understood was gratifying. It was like having proof that I hadn't been making up my symptoms for all those years.

As I met other PECs, I felt an overwhelming need to help them. But how? I believed that I understood how this illness worked and how to recover from it, but I couldn't explain it easily.

I tried to assist one person by sending her to doctors and naturopaths for specific tests. I told her that these would be insightful and that certain treatments would make massive and quick improvements.

She listened eagerly, but did nothing.

She just wanted to talk to me, to share her experience, to be listened to by someone who would not label her a whinger or hypochondriac. She even introduced me to some of her family, to attest that she was not making up her symptoms.

I understood her lack of action: It's treatment exhaustion. I had experienced it long ago myself, when I had given up any hope of recovering. After you have tried so many things and invested so much energy, hope, and money into treatments that fail, you just don't see the point in trying any longer.

Still, I wanted to share my information with other PECs and medical professionals. After I finished my research, it took eighteen months to put it into words. I spent another year sharing it via the Internet. Along the way, I discovered further insights and other researchers who believed in the same hypothesis or important parts of it.

In fact, I used some of my insight to further improve my health and fitness regimen, when I never thought I would be talking about a fitness regimen again.

I've decided that the best way to share my knowledge is to let you follow my trail of discovery. Along the way you'll come to understand important medical concepts that will help you to recover.

As I've said before, this book is not a medical text, scientific proof, or exhaustive examination of my concepts. It shares my explanation for CFS, with enough supporting information to give you confidence in it, and with a framework for recovery.

In my opinion, *the most important aspect of recovery is correcting the central cause of CFS*, in conjunction with treating the secondary problems. I have tried my best not to labour on about details that you can easily get from other books or from your doctor or naturopath. In fact, as your body heals, many of the secondary problems will resolve themselves. If any of them don't, you should seek advice from a doctor or naturopath or draw on one of the many books that cover the problem.

You'll have the best chance of grasping the technical parts of this book if you read it in order. At times, you may feel overwhelmed by the terminology and complexity and not understand everything. That's okay. You will still get enough of the big picture to become the manager of your good health.

Like the owner of a large company, you don't need to understand every detail yourself; you can hire others to help you. Don't try to become a doctor, naturopath, endocrinologist, microbiologist, or biochemist. Just become streetwise enough to hire the right people to help you get your health back.

Most important is that you actually do what needs to be done. Nobody else can do that for you. I can't emphasise this enough. I understand how hard this may be, but you cannot simply hand over the responsibility for your recovery to someone else. You must always decide what is right for you, take whatever actions are needed, and accept any outcome as being a result of your decisions. Only then can you be truly empowered.

You can beat this.

With love, I wish you the best of health and an early recovery.

Dan Neuffer

Chapter Summary

- This book does not replace medical advice. Your treatments should be supervised by a skilled medical doctor. You must receive a diagnosis of CFS from a doctor rather than being self-diagnosed, to ensure that you don't have another illness that requires a different treatment.

- This book deals with a spectrum of conditions that may be known by the following names:

  - Chronic Fatigue Syndrome (CFS),
  - Myalgic Encephalomyelitis (ME),
  - Fibromyalgia or Fibromyalgia Syndrome (FMS),
  - Systemic Exertion Intolerance Disease (SEID),
  - Postural Orthostatic Tachycardia Syndrome (POTS),
  - Chronic Fatigue and Immune Dysfunction Syndrome (CFIDS),
  - Multiple Chemical Sensitivity (MCS),
  - Electromagnetic Hypersensitivity (EHS)
  - Post-Viral Fatigue Syndrome (PVFS).

In this text, all these illnesses are identified as Chronic Fatigue Syndrome (CFS).

Other conditions are likely to fall along the same spectrum of illness, but include specific triggers and secondary dysfunctions that make them more uniquely identifiable. These include the following:

  - Gulf War Syndrome (GWS) and
  - Complex Regional Pain Syndrome (CRPS)
  - Reflex Sympathetic Dystrophy Syndrome (RSD)

- This book refers to people experiencing CFS as PECs.

- To get the fullest understanding of CFS, read this book in order and do not skip ahead.

- Few texts on CFS provide a detailed explanation of its cause. This book is designed to help you understand what causes the illness and what perpetuates it.

continued

- You may feel overwhelmed by the terminology or complexity of this book and not understand everything. That is okay. Just understand enough to gain confidence in the hypothesis and the framework for your recovery.

- You need to take responsibility for your recovery, as only you are able to make it happen.

CHAPTER 5

You Are Not Alone!

"As human beings, we need to know that we are not alone, that we are not crazy or completely out of our minds, that there are other people out there who feel as we do, live as we do, love as we do, who are like us."

- Billy Joel

Exhaustion, fever, pain, swollen throat:
"It's the flu. You'll get over it."

Inability to get out of bed in the morning, stiffness, lethargy:
"You just need to move, get some exercise!"

Smelling strange odours, like ammonia:
"In all my years of medical practice, I've never heard of anything like that."

Asking for help is hard and sometimes disappointing. The problems of CFS are not always visible to outsiders. You may not look sick or have obvious mental dysfunctions, so friends, family, and doctors may not understand or believe you. But consider this: Before you got ill, would you have been able to understand someone experiencing CFS?

Here are some of the common symptoms of CFS:

- **Severe fatigue.** This is not Friday-night-after-a-tough-week tired. You may struggle to walk, lift your arms, or even talk. The fatigue exists at rest but is worsened by activity. It's not like the fatigue of depression, which usually improves when people get out and about.

- **Muscle or joint pain,** more severe than with the flu. The location varies; some people get pain at the back of neck and upper back whilst others may feel pain in the limbs or feet. (With fibromyalgia, pain is the more prominent symptom, as opposed to CFS, where fatigue is more prominent.)
- **Loss of muscle power.** This may come on rapidly or develop over time and it worsens the effects of the fatigue.
- **Loss of mental power,** such as brain fog or memory impairment. You can't think well. This can be upsetting, especially when those around you don't understand. Simple things become difficult, you may get emotional, and you may even find it hard to communicate with people who are not directly in front of you. You may struggle in busy environments like shopping centres or with simple tasks like following a shopping list.
- **Other flu-like or virus-like symptoms,** such as fever, swollen glands, sore throats, headaches.
- **Unrefreshing sleep.** Whilst you may feel sleepy during the day, getting to sleep at night is difficult. You may have a restless feeling, twitchy muscles, or other odd symptoms. When you do sleep, you tend to wake up a lot. In the morning, you feel like you haven't slept and may feel bodily stiffness and pain.
- **Gastrointestinal problems.** PECs seem to be plagued by diarrhoea, constipation, abdominal pain, or bloating, or sometimes all of the above.
- **Infections.** Bacterial, viral, fungal, or parasitic—it's often one after the other, and they often come back.
- **Decreased libido.** It's not just not being in the mood because you are unwell; PECs often show little interest during periods of relative wellness.
- **Multiple chemical sensitivities.** Even a brief exposure to

smoke, pesticides, plastics, scented products, or (in particular) petroleum products and paints may cause strong reactions such as nausea, headaches, fatigue, and other symptoms.

- **Electromagnetic hypersensitivity.** Exposure to mobile phones, base stations, Wi-Fi, or cordless technologies may lead to burning sensations, rashes, concentration losses, headaches, nausea, pains, palpitations, or flu-like symptoms.

Less common symptoms include the following:
- **Orthostatic hypotension,** or the falling of a person's blood pressure as they stand up. You may feel momentarily dizzy or nauseated or have dimmed vision, numbness, or tingling
- **Frequent urination,** along with unquenchable thirst
- **Heart palpitations and chest pains**
- **Muscle twitching,** sometimes described as jolts or flashes
- **Chills and cold extremities**
- **Allergies**
- **Significant weight gain** or loss and loss of muscle mass

You may have psychological symptoms, such as the following:
- **Mood swings**
- **Anxiety**
- **Depression**
- **Irritability**
- **Emotional 'flattening'**

You may also have stranger and more obscure symptoms:
- **Strange smell sensations,** often described as ammonium
- **Allodynia**, when your skin hurts when touched
- **Paresthesia,** or sensations such as itching, numbness, tingling, burning, or the feeling that something is crawling on you
- Hypersensitivity to sound or light
- Profuse sweating
- **Feelings of heat in the body,** especially around the head and neck

It's not surprising that a person with so many diverse symptoms can look like a hypochondriac. MCS, or multiple chemical sensitivities, can seem especially odd. One PEC told me he plans his approach to the petrol station according to the direction of the wind on the day, because the fumes can send him to bed desperately ill for days. It's hard for a healthy person to imagine such a thing, or for a medical doctor to believe it, given that a whiff of petrol has very little toxic load.

The important point is that many other people share your experience. It has been estimated that more than one million Americans and over 250,000 people in the UK have CFS. Worldwide, the figures may be in the tens of millions. **You are not alone!**

Ignorance of CFS and scepticism towards PECs is declining in both the general and medical communities. If you have suffered because of these attitudes, put it behind you as best as you can. If others haven't validated your illness, I hope my words will.

CFS is not your fault. It is not hypochondria and it is not depression. PECs are not weak minded—in fact, research indicates exactly the opposite. Therein lies another clue, which we will discuss later in this book.

CHAPTER 6

The Cause and Conundrum of CFS

"Yet when one suspects that a man knows something about life that one hasn't heard before one is uneasy until one has found out what he has to say."

- Frederick Pollock

Most cases of CFS start suddenly, along with a range of flu-like symptoms. It's like the flu from hell that just won't go away, but over time, the array of symptoms expands.

Researchers have many theories about the cause of CFS. This may be because CFS can have so many different symptoms that just about any dysfunction or illness can explain some of them.

Some studies suggest that CFS is caused by a rare virus (xenotropic murine leukaemia virus-related virus or XMRV), or by more common viruses such as Epstein-Barr, but these theories have not been proven.

Whilst PECs may have many viruses, I believe these are opportunistic and not the cause of the illness. However, viruses and vaccinations can help trigger CFS.

Other theories suggest biochemical dysfunctions as the cause, perhaps because PECs are genetically disposed to them. Biochemical dysfunctions do occur in a large proportion of PECs, and they can explain some of the symptoms. But I don't believe they are the cause of CFS as they don't answer these questions:

Why do some PECs recover quickly and others never recover?

Why do some PECs recover spontaneously?

Why do some PECs recover using the following:

- *Treatments for yeast infections or candida*
- *Treatments for irritable bowel syndrome*
- *Treatments for the adrenals*
- *Treatments to help detoxification*
- *Medication to restore sleep*
- *Medication to restore wakefulness*
- *Medication to make you feel happier*
- *Medication to kill viral infections*
- *Medications to kill bacterial infections*
- *Medications to kill parasites and other infections*
- *Medications to reduce pain*
- *Vitamin supplements*
- *Mineral supplements*
- *Special diets*
- *Meditation and relaxation*

Why do other PECs use these treatments but not recover?

Most of the medical research into CFS explains a lot of the symptoms and dysfunctions, but doesn't ask the most important question.

It's the question that tested the patience of my school teachers. It's the question that challenged my university lecturers and fellow students. It's the question that saved my life.

Why?

Part Two:
Unravelling CFS

CHAPTER 7

Starting with What We Know

"Although Darwin was able to persuade much of the world that a modern eye could be produced gradually from a much simpler structure, he did not even attempt to explain how the simple light sensitive spot that was his starting point actually worked."

- Michael Behe

After reviewing the literature on CFS, I decided that the most logical place to start my research was by listing what we know:

- The most common dysfunctions and symptoms of CFS
- The vitamin and mineral deficiencies PECs have, and the supplements that have some positive impact
- The occurrence of certain trigger events at the onset of the illness

PECs often have different symptoms and dysfunctions, so I decided to start my investigation with what we have in common, the second and third items on the list above; the vitamin and mineral deficiencies, and triggers at the onset of CFS.

Starting with What We Know

CHAPTER 8

The First Clue: Deficiency and the Energy Crisis

S tudies show that vitamins and minerals—most notably B vitamins and magnesium—are low in PECs. Supplements cause notable improvements but not cures.

So I asked myself:

How are these substances used in the body?

Why would PECs have too little of them?

In fact, they are used everywhere in our cells to create energy.

How do our bodies create energy?

Every cell in our bodies needs energy to keep it alive and functioning well. The energy comes from of a molecule called adenosine tri-phosphate (ATP). Think of this molecule as the energy currency in the body.

Our bodies use energy for everything, like contracting the muscles that make our hearts beat. With each such action, ATP gets used up and so our bodies need a constant supply of ATP. No ATP, no life.

So let's take a closer look at ATP in Figure 1, What Is ATP?

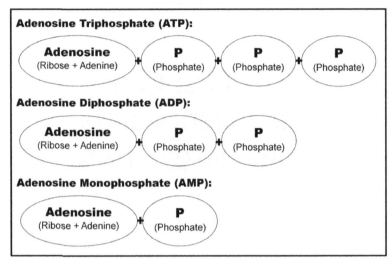

Figure 1: What is ATP?

ATP is made up of a molecule called adenosine with three phosphate ions attached, hence the name adenosine tri-phosphate.

When I said above that "ATP gets used up," I meant that the chemical energy of one of the three phosphate ions gets used up. A phosphate ion is lost. This reduces ATP (adenosine **tri**-phosphate) to ADP (adenosine **di**-phosphate). The ADP is then recycled by the body and turned back into ATP.

The body contains around 200 grams of ATP and ADP. That's not a lot. But it may use a couple of hundred kilos of ATP in a day. This means these molecules must be recycled hundreds of times a day.

Most of this happens in a process called aerobic cell respiration, via the Krebs cycle (also called the citric acid cycle). This leads into a process called oxidative phosphorylation. I will explain this in more detail later, but for now just know that these processes need oxygen.

We only have enough energy in our bodies to last a short period of time. So what happens if due to exercise, illness, or some other stressor, we need more energy than we have available?

Consider Figure 2, ATP Degeneration and Recycling.

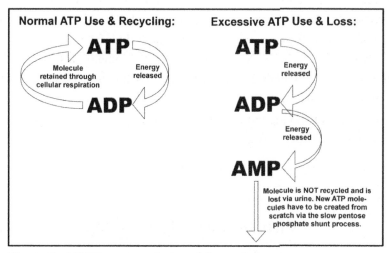

Figure 2: ATP Degeneration and Recycling

If the body needs more ATP than it has available, it will first use a process called lactic acid fermentation. This is what happens when we run until our legs ache. The aching feeling is lactic acid build up. It appears that PECs suffer from chronic lactic acid in the body which causes a lot of the physical pain and symptoms. Some people say this is the cause of fibromyalgia pain. (I'll say more about this later.)

But if we still need more energy, we can use the unrecycled ADP. This is done via the myokinase reaction, which uses up one of the two remaining phosphate ions. This turns ADP (adenosine **di**-phosphate) into AMP (adenosine **mono**-phosphate).

The problem with this is that AMP is not easily recycled. Instead, it is largely lost via urine.

Now your body must make ATP from scratch. This is a long, slow process!

How slow? A Swedish study found that a group of men exercising intensely twice a day for one week had a 25% drop in ATP levels. Even after three days of rest, levels were still down by over 19%. That's in a healthy body.

Once we are overtaxed, then, it takes time to get back to normal.

Nature designed us to work within certain limits, a certain 'energy envelope'. We can exceed it for short periods—say three minutes, or maybe an hour to some extent—but we can't do it for months.

Every process in the body needs energy. Coping with stressors like illness requires even more energy than we usually use. This overtaxing of the body can explain PECs' ATP deficits, their energy crises, and the importance of staying within their body's energy envelope.

However, the question remains:

Why does the energy crisis in PECs never end?

Mitochondrial dysfunction

Because we need ATP to survive, different systems work together to create it or to recycle it from ADP.

To simplify my explanation, I'll ignore two systems for short-term energy needs. Instead, I'll focus on two other pathways, (a) cellular respiration, which creates most of our energy by recycling ADP back into ATP, and (b) lactic acid fermentation, which I mentioned above.

You don't have to understand everything in this section, but it's important to understand the different results of the two pathways.

The pathways are shown in Figure 3, Glucose Metabolism: Recycling ADP into ATP. Protein, fat, and carbohydrates break down into glucose (also known as blood sugar). The Figure shows how our bodies use that glucose to create energy.

The first step in both pathways is **anaerobic respiration** (meaning respiration without oxygen, also called glycolysis). This process is inefficient and creates only about two ATP molecules, as well as two pyruvate molecules.

Normally, our bodies follow the left pathway, cellular respiration, and next perform **aerobic respiration** (respiration with oxygen). Aerobic respiration uses the two pyruvate molecules and oxygen in two stages, the Krebs cycle and a process called oxidative phosphorylation. This creates roughly a further thirty-four ATP molecules. So our cells create thirty-four ATP molecules with oxygen but only two without. That's why we need oxygen to live.

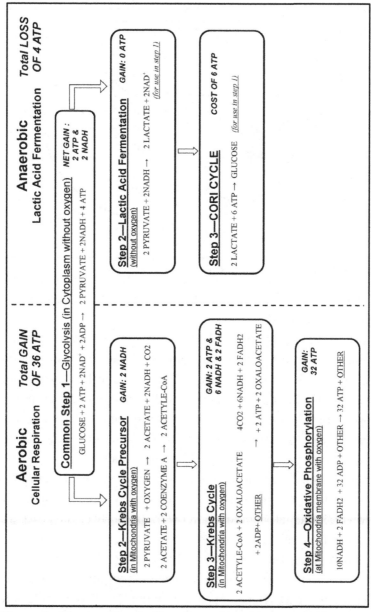

Figure 3: Glucose Metabolism: Recycling ADP into ATP

Let's look at Figure 4, Basic Cell Structure, to see where these processes happen.

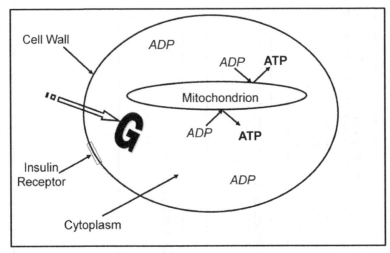

Figure 4: Basic Cell Structure

Around the outside of the cell is a cell wall. Certain doors in this wall let in glucose (the big G).

The space inside the cell is called the cytoplasm. Anaerobic respiration (the first step in both pathways) takes in the cytoplasm.

In the cytoplasm are smaller structures called mitochondria (singular: mitochondrion), much smaller and more plentiful than shown here. The two stages of aerobic respiration happen here. The Krebs cycle occurs inside the mitochondria and oxidative phosphorylation occurs at the walls of the mitochondria.

Since aerobic respiration produces far more molecules of ATP, the mitochondria are where most of our energy production happens. However, if the mitochondria don't work properly or the process fails for any reason, then anaerobic respiration takes over. This is a pretty tough task given that it produces only two ATP molecules.

There's another problem. After anaerobic respiration, molecules of pyruvate and NADH are left in the cytoplasm. If the mitochondria don't take these in for aerobic respiration, they react with each other to produce lactic acid, which brings us to the right pathway in Figure 3, lactic acid fermentation.

This lactic acid causes a range of problems. First, lactic acid in muscle tissue produces the pain and inflammation we experience after exercising. Second, the acidification of our tissue interferes with oxygen supply. This lack of oxygen makes it more difficult for aerobic respiration and the Krebs cycle to start working again.

The body can convert the lactic acid back into glucose via a process called the Cori cycle. The problem is that this process costs six ATP molecules. In other words, anaerobic respiration uses a glucose molecule to make two ATP molecules, then uses six ATP molecules to remake the glucose. **This is a net loss of four ATP molecules.**

Let me go over this again.

Normally, the body makes two ATP molecules via anaerobic respiration, then uses the by-products to make thirty-four more with aerobic respiration, for a total of thirty-six ATP molecules.

If we use only anaerobic respiration, we end up losing four ATP molecules instead.

So that's **a net difference of forty ATP molecules!**

Our cells are supposed to be making energy for use, not draining energy reserves just for survival.

The anaerobic/lactic acid fermentation process works for short-term use. If we use emergency energy to run away from a bear, we can make it up later. **But if that is our primary way of making energy, we are in trouble: We are running an energy deficit.**

And it's even worse than that. Look back at Figure 2, Cellular ATP Degeneration. Not only are we not recycling ADP efficiently to create enough ATP, we don't have enough ADP to recycle, because in the emergency-energy mode, we've been breaking ADP down into AMP. (Remember, AMP is largely lost via urine.)

This means that even if the Krebs cycle suddenly begins working again, we won't have much ADP left for it to recycle into ATP.

Now, the body can get around this. The body can get around just about anything except a lack of essential nutrients.

The body creates new ATP via what is called the pentose phosphate shunt. However, as we mentioned, this process is slow. (Remember the Swedish study that showed ATP deficits of 19% even after three days of recovery.) If we are burning up our ATP faster than we can make it, the energy problem is compounded.

As you saw in Figure 3, aerobic respiration takes place in two stages: the Krebs cycle and oxidative phosphorylation. Let's call these 'the energy reactions' for now.

These energy reactions are essential for creating energy without pain and inflammation. We know there is a problem with these energy reactions in PECs for several reasons:

1. The severe exhaustion suggests that this process is not working properly.
2. Studies have shown elevated levels of lactate in PECs.
3. PECs are known to be often low in magnesium. When they take certain compounds needed for the energy reactions, their CFS symptoms decrease.

The most important compounds for the energy reactions include magnesium, vitamins B1, B2, B3, B5, B6, B7 and B12, manganese, and folic acid. The body can produce some other needed compounds, such as oxaloacetic acid, malic acid, and the enzyme coenzyme Q10 (CoQ10). We also need glucose, oxygen, and water.

The cycle might stop working smoothly because of a lack of these substances. The energy reactions are a complex series in which each step requires the products of earlier reactions plus other compounds. If any of the substances are lacking, the cycle can't continue.

I can suggest several possible reasons for this dysfunction.

1. The ATP shortfall and the subsequent loss of ADP (when it becomes AMP) means ATP needs to be created from scratch.
2. The shutdown of the Krebs cycle may mean that the body isn't making some needed substances, such as oxaloacetic acid. Also, some toxic materials such as acetaldehyde may build up in the body.

3. Evidence shows that glucose (blood sugar) can't get into the cell (due to hypoglycaemia and insulin resistance, which we'll discuss shortly).

4. The highly acidic environment interferes with the cellular oxygen supply, which in turn slows down aerobic respiration.

But questions remain:

Why does mitochondrial dysfunction happen in the first place?

Why does it continue?

Why does it start up again for some people and not for others?

Why do we have all the other symptoms of CFS?

CHAPTER SUMMARY

- PECs often lack the nutrients needed for energy production. Taking supplements of these has a positive impact on PECs.
- The key substances for the energy reactions include:
  - B1
  - B2
  - B3
  - B5
  - B6
  - B7
  - B12
  - Magnesium
  - Manganese
  - Folic acid
  - Coenzyme Q10
  - Oxaloacetic acid
  - Malic acid
  - Oxygen
  - Glucose
  - Water
- Normally, ADP molecules are recycled back into ATP by cellular respiration, which involves both anaerobic and aerobic respiration.
- Aerobic respiration produces most of our energy and happens in two stages. The first is called the Krebs cycle; it occurs inside our mitochondria. The second is called oxidative phosphorylation; it occurs at the walls of our mitochondria.
- A disruption in the Krebs cycle at any point can cause the cycle to stop creating energy. This is because the product from each step of the process is needed for the next step.
- When not enough energy is produced by normal methods, anaerobic respiration/lactic acid fermentation takes over. Whilst this provides extra energy in the short term, it causes an energy deficit.
- Lack of energy, or ATP, can cause the body to draw on ADP. The ADP then turns into AMP, which can't easily be recycled and is lost. This robs the body of ADP needed for recycling into ATP.

CHAPTER 9

The Second Clue:
Onset Trigger Events

"There are very few certainties that touch us all in this mortal experience, but one of the absolutes is that we will experience hardship and stress at some point."

- Dr James C Dobson

D uring my research, I looked at CFS from different angles, including PECs themselves and their experiences when they got sick: Was CFS genetic? Was it caused by an infection? By something PECs did? What I found was at first extremely confusing.

Some people had had glandular fever (mononucleosis caused by the Epstein-Barr virus), something my blood tests showed I'd had. Other people had other infections, flu-like symptoms, and so on.

Some people hadn't had an infection, but they'd had other striking experiences: car accidents, assaults, physical abuse, surgeries, childbirth, vaccinations, a major diet change, or toxic exposures to mould, pesticides, or other poisons.

Others had had more normal but still-intense events: periods of hard physical exercise or study for exams, relationship breakdowns, divorces, abuse at home or at work, job losses, financial pressures, the deaths of loved ones, having to care for someone, or periods of pressure or turmoil due to self-judgment.

The more I looked, the more different events came up. But there was nearly always *something*.

In fact the vast majority of PECs had a period of some kind of turmoil or big event in the twelve to eighteen months before they first got sick. Sometimes it was a physical event like an injury, an infection, child birth or a period of severe exercise. Sometimes it was a psychological upset, like an emotional trauma, a relationship breakdown, the loss of a loved one, or something else that was very upsetting. Most often, it was **multiple stressors of both types**.

These varied experiences all have one thing in common: The body sees them as stress and responds physiologically, through the nervous system and through the endocrine system. The endocrine system releases hormones to help us deal with these challenges, whether they are infections, injuries or psychological experiences that could signal an upcoming physical strain.

But can biological stress cause all these symptoms?

After all, many people have stress yet don't have CFS. And many PECs didn't *feel* stressed before they came down with it.

What is stress?

When we hear the word *stress,* we often think of *feeling* stressed— of mental or emotional stress. But stress can also be physical, and even mental or emotional stresses involve reactions in the body.

Hans Selye, the pioneering endocrinologist who coined the term *stress,* defined it as "the non-specific response of the body to any demand for change." Another definition **defines stress as a response that comes from a gap, real or perceived, between a demand and the ability to meet that demand.** A good example of that gap might be the energy crisis in PECs.

An important thing to realise is that we can be under stress even when we don't *feel* stressed!

A person with an infection may feel tired but otherwise at ease. Athletes in competition may feel joy and exhilaration, but as they push themselves to perform, their bodies are under severe stress.

We suffer from physical stress when we have the flu, break an arm, or don't get enough sleep due to some late night fun watching movies or playing videos games. These kinds of physical stress are often not recognized.

Even mental and emotional stress are not well understood. Mental stress may come from intense study or hard work. Emotional stress may come from worry about a family member or being in a difficult relationship.

Stress may even be due to unresolved issues from earlier in life. When we repress issues rather than deal with them, they can fester. Years later, they may resurface to give us another chance to deal with them.

Stress can also come from positive events like getting married, having a baby, buying a home, or moving, especially when several of these things happen in a short period of time.

Stress can be intense and last for a short time or it can be less intense and last for a long time. Either way, **stress is not only a mental experience; it has effects on the body.**

We know that severe stress can kill. If you put a wild animal in a small cage on a busy street, it will die. But surely stress can't cause all the symptoms of CFS? Can our stress levels really be that severe?

Table 1 shows a list of some events that can create severe stress. You may have experienced one or more of these in the twelve to eighteen months leading up to your first symptoms.

Physical Events	Negative Life Events	Positive Life Events
• Physical Injury; • Surgery; • Child birth; • Puberty; • Infection; • Vaccination; • Other Toxic Exposure; • Excessive exercise; • Lack of sleep; • Major diet change;	• Marriage breakup; • Relationship problems; • Financial pressures; • Loss of loved one; • Excessive demands of caring for a sick person; • Excessive work or study pressures; • Loss of a job;	• Getting married; • Promotion; • Retirement; • Active vacation; • Buying a home; • Having a baby; • Moving home; • New relationship; • Child leaving home; • Business expansion;

Table 1: Examples of Potential Stressors

Putting 'normal' stress into context

Ten thousand years ago, we were all hunter-gatherers; farming didn't exist. Even two hundred years ago, much of the world's population was still hunting and gathering food, or at least relying in part on these activities.

In other words, our lives now are drastically different than the ones for which we evolved. We have less difficulty in obtaining food and shelter, but we get less sleep because we have electric lights and enjoy our electronic screen entertainment. We've moved from working the land to working in factories and offices, which has increased our pace of life and daily pressures. Our connections via mobile phones and the Internet bombard us with demands, some of which we simply cannot meet.

For example, we did not evolve to catch up on replying to e-mails whilst on speaker phone to a client (stress), while the boss messages us for an urgent report (Stress), which is interrupted by another phone call on our mobile (Stress) where we learn that our child has been sent to the principal's office (STRESS). We juggle it all quickly, so that we can squeeze in a lunchtime gym session, so that we can look more like the perfect people on TV (Stress). But whilst we exercise, we wonder how our partner feels about our imperfect body (STRESS) and what our boss thinks about our imperfect children's behaviour or client feedback (STRESS, STRESS, **STRESS!**).

What kind of stress did our bodies evolve to cope with? Well, it's actually something quite similar to what most animals experience.

Palaeolithic hunters encountered severe stress during incidents like a life-threatening attack by a wild animal. However, they experienced this stress for only short periods of time, and relatively rarely, given that they normally lived as part of a group and learned how to avoid these dangers. (Any hunter-gatherer who didn't was quickly removed from the gene pool!) So stress in nature usually lasted only a few minutes. You came across a crocodile, which triggered your fight-or-flight response. Then you either got away, killed the crocodile, or were eaten by it. Whichever way it went, within a few minutes, it was all over.

This short-term stress is called acute stress. Stress that lasts, say, thirty minutes, is called chronic stress.

Think about it: Thirty minutes makes it chronic!

How long were you under stress before CFS?

How much stress have you been under since it started?

Imagine suffering intense mental or emotional stress for a long time, then being hit with a physical stress. The stress can then become overwhelming.

Physical effects of psychological stress

The fight-or-flight response involves the arousal of the **sympathetic nervous system** (SNS). When it's aroused, the adrenal glands sitting on top of our kidneys release the two main stress hormones, **cortisol** and **adrenalin**.

Adrenalin raises our heart rate and blood pressure. It shunts blood away from the brain and digestive organs to our muscles—because if a wild animal is upon you, deep thinking won't help and digestion can wait; you need to fight it or run away.

If the stress ends immediately, the adrenaline quickly disappears from our bodies. Ten minutes later, most of it is gone.

Cortisol, on the other hand, is released more slowly and takes much longer to disappear. It acts as a strong anti-inflammatory and reduces the effects of damage. This keeps our immune system from going crazy when it suddenly has to deal with physical trauma. It makes sure that any injury we suffer in a fight with a crocodile or flight from it doesn't overwhelm us. Because cortisol takes time to act, our bodies release it before we are even sure if damage has occurred. If damage does occur, the body will make even more cortisol, but this early release acts as a kind of insurance.

In the presence of adrenalin, cortisol also helps us form strong memories. You need to remember the details of an encounter with a crocodile so that you avoid repeating the experience. Neurologists call this 'flashbulb memory'.

Stress hormones also perform a few other actions that prepare the body to heal.

First, cortisol limits the ability of glucose (blood sugar) to enter our cells, where—as we've seen—it creates energy. Figure 4 shows glucose entering through certain doors. The key that opens those doors is a hormone called insulin. Insulin lets the glucose into the cells, where it can be converted to energy.

Cortisol helps release glucose into the bloodstream, but it reduces the effectiveness of insulin. This means that less glucose enters the cells; it stays in the bloodstream to be used for healing from trauma.

Second, cortisol also releases amino acids from the muscles. In effect, this reduces the size of the muscles. The amino acids are the building blocks for the protein that makes up our muscles. They are needed to build new muscle and replace any damaged tissue. When the crisis passes, then, our bodies will have everything ready to regenerate.

Third, when cortisol breaks down muscle tissue, we lose nutrients that are needed for the Krebs cycle. This is a potential link between stress and the mitochondrial dysfunction we discussed earlier.

Let me summarise what these two stress hormones do.

Adrenalin:

- raises the heart rate
- raises blood pressure
- shunts blood away from the brain
- shunts blood away from the digestive organs
- shunts blood to the muscles for fighting or fleeing

Cortisol:

- suppresses the immune system and reduces inflammation
- releases glucose to increase blood glucose levels
- reduces the effect of insulin to keep blood glucose levels high
- shuts down the reproductive system
- breaks down muscle tissue
- with adrenalin, helps form 'flashbulb memories'

These two lists sound a little like the effects of CFS, don't they?

Our suppressed immune systems then cause further difficulties.

Immune suppression and physical stress

It's not a mistake that stress depresses the immune system; it's a logical and useful step. It ensures that inflammation does not get out of control and kill us when injury occurs.

However, immune suppression is not meant to go on for long periods of time. Our bodies are designed to deal with stress for short periods—minutes, perhaps hours—but not for days or weeks, and definitely not for years.

Physical stress may be a *result* of the depressed immune system. We've all experienced getting run down and then getting sick. We might become vulnerable to viruses that were dormant in our body, such as herpes or Epstein-Barr. Other physical stressors may be an injury, a surgery, a period of excessive exercise, toxic exposure to a chemical, or childbirth. All these put extra pressure on the immune system; and pregnancy actually increases immune suppression.

Immune suppression would explain the slow recovery from the first symptoms of CFS. In fact, PECs may remember small bouts of fatigue before they came down with full-blown CFS. I only remembered mine long afterwards, as I did not give them any attention at the time.

Other symptoms

We've reviewed the symptom of exhaustion (or producing too little energy). We've seen that the cortisol produced by stress may cause nutrient depletion (which can make it even harder to produce energy) and a depressed immune system. So we can see why we have difficulty recovering from physical stress.

But if eventually the original stressors are gone (or much reduced), if we get enough rest (staying within our energy envelopes), and if we eat well (with extra vitamins and minerals), **why don't we recover?**

And why do we have other symptoms such as the following:

- Digestive dysfunction
- Brain fog
- Sleep disturbance
- Massive pain and inflammation
- Increased thirst
- Decreased libido
- Depression and anxiety
- Cardiac symptoms such as arrhythmia
- Chemical sensitivities
- Allergies

Obviously, CFS isn't just a flu that won't go away because we're stressed out and run down! I had to ask myself:

What else is REALLY going on with CFS?

CHAPTER SUMMARY

- Stress is a non-specific response of the body to any demand for change. It can also be seen as a response to a gap between a demand and the ability to meet that demand.
- Stress can come from:
  - Physical trauma (such as infection, injury, surgery, lack of sleep, toxic exposure, childbirth)
  - Negative life events (such as relationship problems, job loss, financial pressures, death of a loved one, excessive work or study, and so on)
  - Positive life events (such as getting married, buying a home, having a baby, moving)
- Stress can make us vulnerable to infections including viral infections that may have been dormant in our bodies, such as Epstein-Barr, herpes, shingles, and so on.
- In nature, severe stress is usually short-term. We are not built to handle excessive stress for long periods of time.
- Stress releases adrenalin and cortisol which do the following:
  - Shunt blood away from the brain
  - Shunt blood away from digestive organs
  - Shunt blood to muscles
  - Suppress immune system
  - Increase blood glucose levels
  - Reduce effectiveness of insulin
  - Break down muscle tissue
  - Deplete the nutrients in our bodies
- Stress causes immune suppression, which can make it harder to recover from physical stresses.

CHAPTER 10

A Major Realisation: It's Not Just One Problem

*"Sometimes I lie awake at night, and I ask, 'Where have I gone wrong?'
Then a voice says to me, 'This is going to take more than one night."*

- Charlie Brown

The human body is very complex and, as you learn the details of how it works, truly astounding.

Each bodily system has a purpose and they are all interconnected. If one thing is wrong, it will affect something else: If our lungs are not working well, our heart will work overtime. If our stomach doesn't produce enough digestive acid, our small intestine will struggle. In other words, problems cause other problems.

When we are under stress for a long period of time, several systems are affected. Let's look a little more closely at how they work and at how they malfunction with CFS.

Digestive dysfunction

Stress is closely linked to bowel dysfunction. (Most of us know about 'having butterflies in our stomach' when we are nervous.) When we have a fight-or-flight response, the SNS (sympathetic nervous system) moves blood away from the digestive system and interrupts its work.

PECs have problems with their digestive systems, including constipation, irritable bowel syndrome, and diarrhoea. **Irritable bowel syndrome** causes discomfort and can lead to frequent diarrhoea or constipation. Also common are bloating and more severe abdominal pain from a condition known as **spastic colon**.

Constant stress, whether we feel it or not, can make cortisol levels surge and then crash. This makes the immune system lose balance. It becomes overactive, leading to allergies and the production of too many inflammatory chemicals.

Inflammation in the gut is a big problem. It can lead to what is known as a **leaky gut**. In this condition, large molecules (endotoxins and xenobiotics) pass straight from the gut into the bloodstream.

An inflamed gut is less able to absorb nutrients, so PECs can develop nutritional deficiencies. Also, if our digestion does not produce the right amount of acid, we will have trouble breaking down proteins.

Inflammation also hinders the gut's immune function. This allows bacteria, parasites, and candida to take hold.

We don't fully understand how stress causes these symptoms. Many animals, including humans, will empty their bowels, bladders, or stomachs (by vomiting) under extreme stress. This is most likely because it makes them lighter and faster and possibly less appetising. (You may have heard of children peeing themselves when scared or colloquial sayings about fear and bodily functions.)

In short, stress and excessive cortisol cause poor intestinal health, which puts more stress on our bodies: The problem causes more problems!

Glucose regulation and insulin resistance

PECs don't just have difficulty making energy from glucose (blood sugar); they also have significant problems managing glucose levels. This is a significant part of the puzzle to understand how many of the symptoms are created. It is also a clue as to what the root dysfunction that causes CFS actually is. But before we go into this, let's look at how our bodies use different nutrients.

How nutrients are used

We know that the Krebs cycle must function efficiently to provide us with energy. We have seen that we need glucose, oxygen, and other nutrients for it to function well. Now let's look in more detail at how nutrients are used.

Our food provides six basic nutrients:

- Proteins
- Carbohydrates
- Fats
- Vitamins
- Minerals
- Water

The first three, carbohydrates, proteins, and fats, are called the macronutrients. The last three, vitamins, minerals, and water, are all used in the Krebs cycle, as well as in many other processes in the body.

Food also contains fibre or roughage which is not a nutrient. Fibre is the parts of plant foods that cannot be digested and helps to absorb water or remove waste from the body.

Having the right amount of fibre is important in order to have healthy bowel function. It slows digestion and the absorption of carbohydrates and hence reduces the rapid rising in blood glucose levels and the corresponding insulin response that follows a meal.

What happens when we eat the three macronutrients; carbohydrates, protein and fats?

You may be surprised to realise that carbohydrates, proteins, and fats are actually physically similar molecules. To some extent, one can be transformed into the other. All three are made from carbon, hydrogen, and oxygen atoms. They are basically arranged differently, and fats and proteins sometimes contain some other atoms.

Let's look at the three macronutrients in turn.

Carbohydrates

Carbohydrates or carbs are not a structural part of the body unlike protein (which is used to form muscle) or fat.

Carbs are just a form of fuel. All carbs are turned into glucose which is then used as fuel for your cells. Some cells such as brain and nerve cells prefer glucose as fuel. **Remember this, because it will be important later on.**

Proteins

Proteins works a little differently. They are essential for building and repairing the body. Proteins are made up of chains of smaller chemicals called amino acids. About twenty different amino acids, in different combinations, make up the countless proteins available in nature.

Our bodies use two types of amino acids, the essential ones that can only be supplied by food and the non-essential ones that can be made by the body.

Animal products contain all the essential amino acids. Plant proteins usually lack at least one essential amino acid. This is why vegetarians have to combine their foods carefully so that they don't miss out on key nutrients.

When we eat proteins, they are digested and broken down into their separate amino acids. This happens as long as our digestion is working and we are producing enough acid (which is not the case in many PECs).

These amino acids are then used to build new proteins that are the building blocks for muscle cells in the body. They are also used to make a range of substances such as hormones and neurotransmitters as well as for energy.

Energy is made from amino acids by converting proteins to glucose in the liver, with some fat to fuel the process. This also creates by-products called ketones. Ketones can also be used by the body as energy, but unlike glucose and fats, they are not stored. They are used as they are created.

Fats or fatty acids

In my opinion, fats have been somewhat unjustly vilified.

Healthy fats support our bodies in many ways. They have little or no impact on blood glucose levels or insulin levels, and they take a long time to metabolise. Our western diet tends to include too many bad fats and not enough good fats. Increasing fat intake can actually be beneficial for several reasons, and I will go into that in the second part of this book.

Fat metabolism is a little more complicated. Several processes convert fats into fatty acids and ketones, as well as into ATP. These processes occur in the liver and other tissues. **Fatty acids are also metabolised in the mitochondria of cells via the Krebs cycle, just like glucose is.** However, fatty acid metabolism is much slower and steadier than carbohydrate metabolism. Slow and steady sounds good, right?

One reason fats may be vilified is because they are very high in energy. Fats provide nine calories of energy per gram, whereas carbs and protein only provide four. A single triglyceride (a form of fat) will eventually produce 441 ATP molecules compared to the 38 produced from a glucose molecule. You can easily see then, why fat is considered a richer source of energy.

Macronutrient summary

Carbohydrates convert quickly and easily into glucose, which is used for energy. Fats and proteins have other uses besides energy, but when used for energy, they are converted more slowly.

For now, we will focus on carbohydrates because of their direct and rapid impact on blood glucose, which is also the essential fuel for the central nervous system (CNS).

Understanding Glucose Regulation

We make glucose from the food we eat. But the amount of glucose in our bloodstream must be carefully regulated. As with ATP, our blood contains only a small amount of glucose at any one time—roughly a teaspoon. That's about enough to let us watch TV for an hour or do four minutes of moderate physical work.

The rest of our glucose is stored for later use, first in muscle and liver cells. When these sites are full, glucose is turned into fatty acids and stored in our fat cells. Extra glucose must be stored quickly, because high blood sugar can cause immediate problems like feeling tired and weak, being thirsty, and urinating a lot.

Insulin is put out by the pancreas when blood glucose (blood sugar) levels get high. For example, after a meal, our bodies show a rapid rise in blood glucose levels and then a rise in insulin. As we've seen, insulin 'unlocks the doors' to let glucose into the cells where it can be used for energy. It also helps store excess glucose in fat and liver cells.

Figure 5 shows a range of blood sugar levels, from too low to too high, and seven pathways by which it may be regulated.

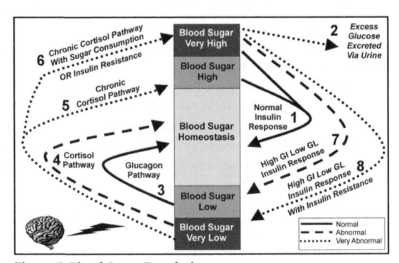

Figure 5: Blood Sugar Regulation

Blood sugar levels are ideal when they are in the middle area, between 4.5 and 5.5 mmoles/l. A healthy body is very good at keeping blood sugar levels within this range.

If blood sugar rises beyond 5.5, the pancreas puts more insulin into the bloodstream. The insulin removes the excess glucose and places it into fat and liver cells. This is the solid line; **Pathway 1**.

If blood sugar continues to rise, to around 8, the kidneys produce more urine to expel the excess blood sugar, as shown in the dotted line; **Pathway 2**. (This is why some diabetics have to urinate a lot and then become thirsty; it may also explain in part why some PECs do the same.)

But **PECs often have hypoglycaemia, in which blood sugar drops too low.** If blood sugar falls to below 4.6, insulin levels decrease.

Below 3.8, the pancreas releases a hormone called glucagon, which has an anti-insulin effect. This is shown in the solid line; **Pathway 3**.

It causes the liver to release glucose into the bloodstream. Adrenaline and growth hormone levels also increase to help raise glucose levels.

If blood sugar levels fall below 3.2, the body will perceive this as a stressful emergency. The adrenal glands then release cortisol. (Once again, we find stress and cortisol, which are common to PECs at the onset of CFS.) This process, shown in the dashed line; **Pathway 4**. It promotes the breakdown of fats and proteins in the body and causes the liver to produce more glucose. Blood sugar levels rise again.

Now the body will react severely to stop a drop in blood sugar levels. It wants to pump out as much anti-insulin glucagon and cortisol as it needs. This keeps the liver busy, but if it's already busy (say, trying to get rid of toxins absorbed via a leaky gut), blood sugar can continue to drop.

When blood glucose levels fall to 2.8, confusion sets in. The brain won't function properly. We become confused, and thinking becomes difficult. Sound familiar?

Unfortunately, **if cortisol is always high, then the body's response to low blood sugar may overshoot its target,** following the dotted

Pathway 5. It can then push blood sugar from too low to too high.

When we feel a drop in energy, we may want to eat a food that converts quickly to blood sugar, such as candy, white bread, pasta, or rice. Then our blood sugar levels quickly spike, as shown in dotted **Pathway 6.** But whilst this may make us feel better at first, we pay a big price for it. Food that converts quickly into glucose usually gets used up quickly, especially if it's only a small snack.

Here's what happens: Feeling hungry, we eat a candy bar. As our blood sugar rises, we need more insulin, so the pancreas stops making the anti-insulin glucagon. As blood sugar spikes, it goes into overdrive, dumping insulin into the bloodstream. Since high blood sugar levels can be very damaging, it will continue to dump in insulin until these levels return to normal.

But the candy bar gives us a blood sugar spike—quick rise, quick fall—so sugar stops entering the bloodstream abruptly. This happens long before the level of sugar already in the bloodstream falls, and long before the pancreas slows down insulin production. By the time it does slow down, the bloodstream contains way too much insulin, and we have a sharp drop in blood sugar. This is shown in **Pathway 7** as the abnormal dashed pathway leading to low blood sugar. If we have severe insulin resistance, the very abnormal pathway leading to very low blood sugar is shown by the dotted **Pathway 8.**

The body sees this low blood sugar as a stress and dumps in cortisol to keep us alive and increase blood sugar. But in PECs, this response is amplified, and so of course, the whole blood sugar roller coaster starts again.

Now another factor comes into play. **Our bodies are designed to stay in balance (homeostasis), so constantly high levels of insulin are countered by something called insulin resistance.**

Remember that insulin is the key that lets glucose through the cell 'doors'. If insulin levels are constantly high, too much glucose comes in, which is not good for the cells. So the cells in effect 'nail some of the doors shut'.

The problem is that when we eat a sugary snack (like the candy bar), the insulin works even more slowly. In the panic to reduce the spike in glucose levels, then, the pancreas pumps out more insulin, and insulin levels overshoot even more. (See dotted **Pathway 6** again.)

Many PECs experience this dynamic. It's a milder version of what happens with Type 2 diabetes or pre-diabetes, or with hypoglycaemia.

These dysfunctions may not show up on a blood glucose test or even a glucose tolerance test (where blood sugar is measured immediately before consuming a sugary drink and then one hour later). Often only a five-hour glucose tolerance test will show the problem, but even that won't necessarily do so. This is because, unlike with Type 2 diabetes or hypoglycaemia, **PECs' blood glucose intolerance is inconsistent**: It doesn't always occur under the same circumstances.

The following is a list of symptoms of hypoglycaemia. (Note that not all of these manifest in every case.)

- Shakiness
- Sweating
- Anxiety and nervousness
- Palpitations and tachycardia
- Coldness and clamminess
- Paresthesia (numbness or a feeling of 'pins and needles')
- Severe hunger
- Headaches
- Nausea and vomiting
- Abdominal discomfort
- Moodiness and exaggerated concerns
- Depression and negativism
- Staring, glassy look
- Anger and irritability
- Fatigue and weakness
- Confusion, delirium, and amnesia
- Flashes of light in the field of vision
- Difficulty speaking, including slurred speech

Once again, this sounds a lot like CFS. In fact, some might suggest that hypoglycaemia causes CFS because of the overlap in symptoms. **The overlap in symptoms between CFS and other illnesses is why it's important to be properly diagnosed with CFS.** However, hypoglycaemia in PECs is a **result**, not a cause, of CFS.

There's another important point about glucose regulation and stress. Whilst adrenaline from stress raises our blood sugar and stimulates our nervous system, it has only a short half-life. (A half-life is how long it takes for the levels to halve.) Adrenaline lasts for five minutes or so in our blood. Cortisol, on the other hand, has a half-life of around eighty minutes. That is, after eighty minutes, fifty percent of the cortisol remains, and after 160 minutes, twenty-five percent remains. **If we are under repeated stress, we will have continuously high levels of cortisol.**

Over time, the cycle of stress leads to chronically high insulin and cortisol levels as well as insulin resistance. By 'chronically high', I don't mean high at every moment; I mean high on average over a period of time, say twenty-four hours or even a week. This can happen even if you are eating a relatively good diet, or a diet that's not any worse than many other people who don't have CFS.

This raises other questions, such as why PECs under- and overshoot their blood glucose levels. That's an important question and one that will lead us to the primary cause of CFS in this hypothesis. But for now, let's follow the thread of cortisol and dysfunctions in the body.

Cortisol Dysregulation

Cortisol and Sympathetic Nervous System (SNS) arousal came up when we spoke about stress at the onset of CFS.

Cortisol and SNS arousal came up when we spoke about gut dysfunction.

Cortisol and SNS arousal came up when we spoke about hypoglycaemia and blood sugar regulation.

What is all this talk about cortisol and the SNS?

First, let me back up a little and introduce the **Autonomic Nervous System (ANS)**. The ANS is part of our Central Nervous System (CNS) and works mainly subconsciously. It controls involuntary functions such as blood pressure, heartbeat, breathing, and digestion. Its main purpose is to help us deal with the demands placed on us, which means that it responds to all stressors, both physiological ones (like hard physical labour, infection or injury) as well as psychological stressors and emotions. It can be divided into two subsystems, the sympathetic and parasympathetic nervous systems.

The Sympathetic Nervous System (SNS), which we've mentioned, controls the body's response to danger. It prepares the body for 'fight or flight' by increasing heart rate, breathing, and perspiration, by slowing digestion, and by dilating the pupils.

The Parasympathetic Nervous System (PNS) balances the SNS by helping to calm the body when it's out of danger.

The hypothalamus in the brain is part of the ANS. It connects to the endocrine (hormonal) system via the pituitary gland.

To understand how this works, let's look at Figure 6, which shows the hypothalamus in the brain and its role in regulating stress hormones.

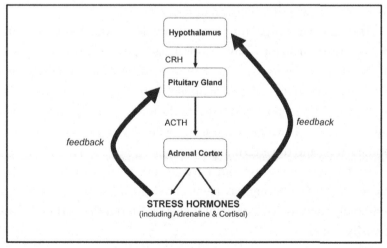

Figure 6: Stress Hormone Regulation

When we are under stress, the SNS takes over. The hypothalamus releases a hormone called Corticotrophin-Releasing Hormone (CRH) to stimulate the pituitary gland.

The pituitary gland is called the master gland because it controls the function of the other endocrine glands. If we look at even one part of it—the anterior lobe—it releases not only adrenocorticotropic hormone (ACTH) and growth hormone, but also hormones to stimulate the adrenals, the thyroid gland, and the ovaries and testes, among other things. **So any dysfunction of the pituitary gland may potentially affect every hormone and system in the body.** Does that sound significant to you?

The pituitary produces ACTH. ACTH tells the adrenals to release dozens of different hormones, but the main ones are the following:

- DHEA (5 dehydroepiandrosterone), used to make sex hormones such as testosterone, estrogens, and progesterone
- Aldosterone, which regulates sodium–potassium balance to control blood pressure as well as a number of other functions
- Cortisol, which counteracts insulin, raises blood glucose levels, and has a number of other effects

Adrenaline is also released during stress, but this response is much faster than the cortisol response. As we've seen, cortisol levels rise with stresses, whether physical or psychological.

The normal range for cortisol levels in the body is usually between 20 and 50 mg a day. Levels usually peak in the morning, when blood sugar reserves are at their lowest. At this time, the body produces cortisol in order to maintain blood sugar levels and wake us up. Cortisol then steadily decreases during the day, with a couple of smaller upwards swings at the times when we tend to get hungry, in midmorning and the afternoon.

Under extreme stress, our cortisol levels can go much higher. A range of 200 to 500 mg has been noted. In other words, **stress can massively increase our cortisol levels, up to ten times their normal, healthy range.**

Why would cortisol levels be chronically up?

First, we know about the stress at the onset of CFS.

Second, a poor diet, which causes high blood sugar, and the elevated stress levels of our western lifestyle can also cause high cortisol— which in turn causes high blood sugar, creating a cycle. (This goes part of the way to explain why so many people in our society lack energy and depend on coffee, sugar, and other stimulants to get through the day.)

As I've explained, cortisol counteracts insulin and raises blood sugar levels. Our cells have to adapt by responding less to insulin and 'nailing the doors shut' to blood sugar. When this happens, we need higher levels of insulin to get blood sugar into the cells, but **insulin is very inflammatory.**

In order for the body to function well, it uses many feedback mechanisms. The hypothalamus and pituitary gland sense cortisol levels and regulate them appropriately. In the short term, when cortisol levels are high, some of the cortisol receptors are shut off. This means we need higher levels of cortisol before we reduce the production of CRH and ACTH.

This makes sense if we put it into caveman terms. If you are in an ongoing stressful situation—say, a bear visits your group's cave each night to eat one of your tribe—you don't want to decrease your ability to produce cortisol. You want to maintain enough capacity until the situation ends, even if it makes you feel a little run down and sleepless.

However, eventually the feedback cycles will down-regulate to lower the amount of stress hormones created. This is because, regardless of the situation, **your cortisol levels need to come down.**

This happens because high cortisol levels are very damaging. Cortisol and other stress hormones suppress the immune system and interfere with important bodily functions such as digestion. If the stress response persists for a long time, the ANS must down-regulate it.

Adrenal insufficiency/adrenal fatigue

Too much cortisol and other adrenal hormones are bad for the body. However, a lack of these hormones also creates many symptoms of ill health. It's called **adrenal insufficiency** or adrenal fatigue.

Most doctors don't recognize or treat adrenal insufficiency. However, it is usually a problem for PECs who have been sick for longer periods of time. Some PECs may have had a mild version of it before they were struck down with CFS.

Adrenal insufficiency is a lowered functioning of the adrenal glands. (The technical term for it is hypoadrenia.) The lowered output can be anywhere from just under optimal to nearly nothing. At the 'nearly nothing' end, the medical community makes a diagnosis of Addison's disease, which is very rare. Unfortunately, most MDs see other lower levels of cortisol as normal and healthy. But the human body is not a binary system. Things aren't either working or not working; there is a spectrum of function.

Holistic medical doctors and alternative health care professionals take a different view. They believe that a prolonged period of stress and the massive amounts of cortisol it requires eventually **exhaust** the adrenal glands. The adrenal glands then do not make sufficient adrenal hormones. However, **I believe that the adrenals are not necessarily exhausted but that the body lowers their output for a reason.** That's why I prefer the term 'adrenal insufficiency' to the more common 'adrenal fatigue'.

Adrenal insufficiency is often cited as the cause of CFS. I think it is fair to say that it is a cause *of lots of the symptoms* of CFS.

Here are some of the symptoms of adrenal insufficiency:

- Excessive fatigue and exhaustion
- Non-refreshing sleep (difficulty getting up in the morning)
- A feeling of being overwhelmed by or unable to cope with stressors
- A craving for salty foods
- A craving for sweet foods

- A crash in energy in the afternoon around 4 pm, feeling most energetic in the evening after dinner, followed by sleepiness around 9-10 pm, then a second wind around 11 pm-1 am
- Lightheadedness when standing up quickly
- Less focussed, fuzzy brain or memory problems
- Mild depression, high irritability, and moods swings
- Very strong premenstrual syndrome (PMS) in women
- Decreased sex drive
- Frequent sighing
- Sensitivity to cold and feeling chilled
- Decreased ability to recover from illness

Sound like CFS, doesn't it?

Not surprisingly, people with adrenal insufficiency also often suffer from hypoglycaemia. But not all PECs have adrenal insufficiency, especially at the onset of CFS.

Whilst treating adrenal insufficiency works for some PECs, it doesn't work for many others. **In fact, treating adrenal insufficiency will make many PECs feel worse or cause them to relapse, since they will begin to feel the effects of high levels of cortisol again.**

The adrenal glands can even atrophy or shrink over time. My research leads me to believe that this may have to do with the reduced output of ACTH, which I believe acts as a growth hormone for the adrenal gland. Without this stimulation, the adrenals shrink.

If you push yourself hard enough, you can most likely squeeze out a short burst of adrenal hormones. You might do this by getting angry or using other emotions to stimulate yourself. This allows you to go from sluggish to capable for a short time, but afterwards you will crash and find yourself in worse shape than before.

Other hormonal and neurotransmitter dysfunctions

Other substances besides adrenal hormones show lower-than-normal levels or other dysfunctions in CFS. They include the following:

- Thyroid hormone, which regulates metabolism
- Melatonin, a hormone which regulates the body's circadian rhythm to help with sleep
- Serotonin, an important neurotransmitter affecting mood and closely linked with depression
- Testosterone and estrogens, which are sex hormones with a wide variety of functions

The lowered levels of these hormones can be explained in a variety of ways, but it's mostly because regulation and production is shared via both the adrenal and pituitary glands.

If you look at the symptoms these low levels cause, you will again get a list similar to CFS symptoms. However, they are secondary problems and not the primary cause of CFS.

Immune dysfunction

This is primarily another effect of too much and too little cortisol, but it's worth looking at separately.

When we have too much cortisol in our bloodstream, it depresses our immune system. That is why people feel run down after they've been under too much stress, whether it is physical or psychological stress.

Excessive cortisol can hinder the white blood cells that make up the immune system from maturing. Cortisol also suppresses the release of the interleukin messengers, which make these white blood cells less responsive.

All this happens in the thymus gland, and over time, cortisol can cause the thymus gland to shrink. If that isn't bad enough, cortisol can even kill white blood cells by destroying their DNA.

No wonder PECs are susceptible to every stray virus, bacteria, fungus, or parasite.

If all this goes on long enough, the overburdened immune cells can start making mistakes and attacking our own cells. This is autoimmune disease. It is especially a problem with adrenal insufficiency, when too much cortisol suddenly turns into too little, effectively removing the breaks on the immune system and allowing it to become overactive.

So without adequate cortisol we are not much better off, because then the resulting overactive immune system can then lead to allergies and contribute to the triggering of multiple chemical sensitivities.

Toxicity and liver dysfunction

We've seen that a leaky gut allows large molecules to enter the blood stream directly. Our bodies then use strong antibody responses to combat these dangerous foreign materials. This burdens the liver, which has to get rid of these toxins. Some of them may be partially processed and accumulate in the liver and fatty tissue.

This toxic load can lead to stress on the liver, leading to skin rashes and inflammation. Also, our livers may already be busy dealing with two other processes:

- the blood sugar rollercoaster of storing glycogen and releasing glucose
- the conversion of broken-down muscle tissue into glucose

If the liver is overworked, it might not do its job very well, allowing toxins to build up. A lifetime of toxic accumulation from food, the environment, and medication also creates pressure on the liver.

The liver may be struggling for other reasons. Most people have a poor diet that lacks the sulphur-containing foods and amino acids that helps the liver produce antioxidants.

Even with a good diet, if our digestive system is damaged, it won't absorb the nutrients properly, so they will never reach the liver. This becomes a loop, in which poor digestion causes poor antioxidant production, which causes inflammation, which causes poor digestion.

The list of symptoms of liver dysfunction is truly amazing. It covers most CFS symptoms, so some people believe it is the cause of CFS. One thing is clear: good liver function is key for good health.

Other cellular dysfunction

We've discussed mitochondrial dysfunction, but how does it begin? The short answer is something called oxidative stress and loss of the required materials such as magnesium and other minerals during periods of stress.

Biochemist Dr Martin Pall has proposed a NO/OONO (nitric oxide peroxynitrate) cycle theory. It suggests that short-term stressors increase the levels of certain chemicals (nitric oxide and/or superoxide and also their oxidant product peroxynitrate) in the body. These chemicals create a vicious cycle which keeps their levels high and causes a lot of the symptoms of CFS. He lists a large range of supplements that should down-regulate this cycle, and these do include the supplements known to reduce CFS symptoms.

Dr Pall's NO/OONO cycle might also interfere with a process called methylation. Methylation is the process of adding methyl groups to molecules. (A methyl group is a carbon atom with three hydrogen atoms attached.) Methyl groups are essential to life and are involved in a very large number of roles in the body including the following:

- Switching genes on or off
- Breaking down neurotransmitters, such as dopamine
- Breaking down estrogen
- Breaking down adrenalin and noradrenalin
- Breaking down histamine, which is involved in inflammation
- Making adrenaline
- Making acetylcholine
- Making lecithin, which helps move fatty acids to the muscles
- Making carnitine, which helps with fatty acid metabolism
- Making creatine, which is important in the energy reservoir system in our muscles
- Keeping the membranes that surround our cells more fluid, to allow better regulation of minerals like sodium and potassium

A breakdown in methylation could explain a lot of the problems with CFS. It would affect energy production in several ways:

- It would affect the production of CoQ10, which is vital for energy production.
- It would affect glutathione production, and without this major detoxification molecule, oxidative damage could easily occur and lead to mitochondrial dysfunction.
- It would cause problems with the creatine phosphate system (the first source of energy our body uses, not discussed in this book), which would burden our other energy systems.
- It would have an effect on carnitine, which is critical in fatty acid metabolism, which would also affect energy.

So too little methylation—hypomethylation—creates energy and detoxification issues. It also impacts the production and metabolism of important hormones and neurotransmitters, a key area of CFS dysfunction. Another problem is the inability to break down histamine. High levels of histamine can trigger inflammation and cause agitation, irritability, and sleep cycle disturbance.

In my opinion, then, hypomethylation can explain a large proportion of the CFS symptoms.

During my research on CFS, I looked at other conditions with similar symptoms, such as autism. This led me to the great work of Dr Amy Yasko, an expert in molecular biology. Her work is groundbreaking, and she is revered by parents of children with autism the world over. What surprised me was that she had worked with CFS as well.

Following this trail, I came across the theories and papers of Dr Richard Van Konyenburg, who passed away in 2012.

Dr Van Konyenburg was a kind man with about thirty years of experience in physics and chemistry who'd dedicated himself to helping people who were suffering from CFS. He proposed that there is a partial block in PECs' methylation cycles. He explained its mechanism and how it causes a large range of symptoms and proposed some supplementation to help correct it.

Medical doctor Neil Nathan performed a trial of Dr Konyenburg's supplementation with the assistance of Dr Amy Yasko's laboratory.

The results were very positive, with significant improvements in the health of the participants as measured by both questionnaires and levels of glutathione and SAMe (a molecule indicating successful methylation).

However, it is important to note that some serious negative results have also been observed since that study and that many PECs have had poor or no results with this treatment.

In my opinion, Dr Van Konyenburg's glutathione depletion theory has correctly identified an important dysfunction in many PECs. His papers describe the dysfunctions and symptoms from a biochemical point of view as opposed to a bodily-system point of view and appear very sound. However, I do not believe this to be root problem of the illness but rather a secondary dysfunction.

I felt the question had to be asked;

What causes the NO/ONOO cycle or breakdowns in glutathione production or methylation?

The answer is oxidative stress, caused by glutathione depletion, caused by excessive stress hormones such as cortisol and adrenaline.

Pain

PECs experiences with pain vary. Some don't experience pain at all, and those who do, experience many sorts of pain. Certain types of pain can lead to a diagnosis of fibromyalgia.

People diagnosed with Fibromyalgia Syndrome will usually have painful tender points that elicit pain when pressure is applied. The criteria has historically required eleven of eighteen tender points to be present in order for this diagnosis to be made.

However, in my view somebody experiencing the many varied symptoms of the **syndrome** and nine or ten of these tender points shouldn't be left undiagnosed. Because if fatigue or orthostatic intolerance isn't part of their range of symptoms (for ME/CFS or POTS diagnosis), they may be left without any diagnosis at all.

Pain is not restricted to just tender points or trigger points which refer pain (often diagnosed as myofascial pain syndrome). PECs also experience migraines, other severe headaches, pain and aches akin to what people get when they have a flu as well as neuropathic pain and allodynia where even the lightest touch on the skin is unbearable.

It has also been shown that PECs experience elevated levels of white blood cells and C-reactive Protein (CRP) which is a marker of increased inflammation in the body.

We also know that levels of certain chemicals involved in pain sensing (substance P) are higher than in healthy people.

Also, it is increasingly recognised that the chronic pain PECs feel is affected by a process called central sensitisation. In this process, the brain learns to feel excessive pain.

Why is all this happening?

It's not hard to see why PECs would experience inflammation, given the large range of their dysfunctions, including problems with the immune system. But the elevated levels of substance P and the central sensitisation process clearly point, once again, towards a central nervous system dysfunction.

A final note

At this point, you may be struggling to understand some of the ideas presented so far, or you might feel that you have read some of them before. In either case, don't worry. Simply keep reading and try to grasp the essence of what is being explained.

We are about to unravel it all.

CHAPTER SUMMARY

- Stress and nervous system dysfunction is involved in many bodily dysfunctions including:
  - Digestive dysfunctions such as leaky gut and irritable bowel syndrome (IBS)
  - Glucose regulation problems and insulin resistance
  - Excessive cortisol levels
  - Adrenal insufficiency
  - Other hormone dysfunctions
  - Immune system dysfunction
  - Toxic build-up and liver dysfunction
  - Pain perception
- Other cellular dysfunctions, such as the proposed NO/ONOO cycle and a possible methylation cycle dysfunction, can also be triggered by stress and also cause many symptoms if they exist.
- In addition to being self-perpetuating, many of these problems interact and perpetuate each other.

CHAPTER 11

A Plausible Hypothesis?

"To believe in something not yet proved and to underwrite it with our lives: it is the only way we can leave the future open. Man, surrounded by facts, permitting himself no surmise, no intuitive flash, no great hypothesis, no risk, is in a locked cell. Ignorance cannot seal the mind and imagination more surely."

- Lillian Smith

The dysfunctions we've discussed so far can explain most of our CFS symptoms. To help you understand this more easily, let's summarise these one by one.

Cortisol from the initial stress eventually can lead to excessive cortisol levels and adrenal insufficiency. The immune system, depressed at first by periods of high cortisol, can then become overactive due to low cortisol leading to inflammation and pain.

Although the immune system is no longer depressed, that does not mean it is working well. We may still be **unable to recover from infections,** which can explain many symptoms of CFS.

The **initial stress** can also affect our gut function, leading to intestinal symptoms such as bloating, constipation, and diarrhoea. These dysfunctions and the depressed immune system can lead to yeast infections, like candida, and eventually **to ongoing problems like irritable bowel syndrome and leaky gut syndrome.** These in turn increase nutritional deficiencies and toxic exposure.

Adrenal insufficiency and other dysfunctions lead to **other low**

hormone production. Symptoms include **sweating, cold extremities, low sex drive, and so on.** Low thyroid hormone levels alone go a long way towards explaining these symptoms.

Hypoglycaemia explains many remaining CFS symptoms. **Excess thirst and urination** can be explained by the body losing fluid from trying to lower high blood sugar. They can also be from an imbalance in our salt–potassium levels from low adrenal hormones. Without enough salt, drinking more may make the problem worse, as it can help wash more minerals, including magnesium, out of the body.

Hypoglycaemia can explain some of the **fatigue.** Even without mitochondrial dysfunction, we know that low blood sugar means low energy. Many neurological symptoms, such as **brain fog, a lack of concentration, and confusion,** are to a large extent explained by low blood sugar.

Some researchers suggest that **inflammation, stiffness, and muscle pain** are caused by **excessive insulin,** since insulin is a powerful inflammatory hormone. Stiffness can come from **low magnesium levels** due to stress and possibly even poor gut function. Low cellular energy due to mitochondrial dysfunction can cause pain in muscle tissue. **Too little cortisol** to balance the inflammation response can bring on more **pain and inflammation.**

Alcohol or chemical intolerance and other failures to cope with toxic burdens can be explained by **liver dysfunction.** The liver is the largest organ in the body. Poor liver function can apparently explain just about anything.

Oxidative stress during the initial period of stress can elevate certain chemical levels leading to the NO/ONOO cycle. It can also **lead to too little methylation,** which in turn can affect our ability to reduce inflammation, make important neurotransmitters, create detoxifying molecules, and ensure efficient fatty acid metabolism, **leaving us with hormone deficiencies, inflammation, more oxidative stress, and a reliance on glucose for energy.**

In other words, we have many explanations for the dysfunctions of CFS, how they are interconnected, and how they cause a large range of symptoms. Perhaps you have heard some of this before.

So many practitioners see CFS exactly this way—as an interlinked collection of dysfunctions that self-perpetuates. They treat the different problems with combinations of naturopathic, nutritional, supplemental, and drug treatments with varying levels of success.

The body is a system, so poor performance in one area affects other areas. We can easily make the case that all these dysfunctions trigger each other and interact. But in my view, **these theories of what causes CFS simply do not add up.** At this point, another quotation comes to mind:

> "In order to shake a hypothesis, it is sometimes not necessary to do anything more than push it as far as it will go."
>
> *- Denis Diderot*

If we push on this reasoning, we still have questions:

Why, when PECS treat one or more of their secondary dysfunctions, do some recover whilst others don't?

If it is just a matter of fixing all the dysfunctions, why do PECs so often relapse?

Why are PECs' recoveries so fragile? Healthy people do not fall easily into this multisystem dysfunction, so why do recovered PECs fall so easily *back* into it?

Clearly, these multisystem explanations do not give us the full answer. However, we shouldn't totally dismiss their merit. They have helped us to explain many of the symptoms of CFS and even a great deal of its self-perpetuating nature. This gives us great insight into steps for recovering from CFS.

The question remains:

What restarts the dysfunctions, even after PECs have broken the self-perpetuating cycles, healed their bodies, and temporarily recovered from CFS?

CHAPTER SUMMARY

- Initial stress can cause several dysfunctions that lead to further problems:

Dysfunctions Due to Stress	Examples of Further Problems Caused by Dysfunctions
Adrenal Excess	Depressed immune system, ongoing infections such as herpes, shingles, Epstein-Barr, even cold and flu
Adrenal insufficiency	Hypoglycaemia, fatigue which can lead to brain fog, inflammation
Hypo-methylation	Excessive histamine, with inflammation and pain; neurotransmitter imbalance and mood disorders, lack of carnitine with impaired fatty acid metabolism and glucose reliance, poor detoxification leading to oxidative stress
Digestive dysfunction	Toxic stress and nutritional deficiencies which can lead to mitochondrial dysfunction
Other hormonal & neurotransmitter dysregulation	Poor temperature regulation, diabetes insipidus, substance P elevation leading to pain increase

- These problems can cause further dysfunctions like autoimmune issues and many others.

- Many of these dysfunctions are self-perpetuating.

- Many of these dysfunctions perpetuate other dysfunctions.

- The question remains:
  What restarts the dysfunctions, even after PECs have broken the self-perpetuating cycles, healed their bodies, and temporarily recovered from CFS?

CHAPTER 12

The Critical Realisation: ANS Dysfunction

"People think of these eureka moments and my feeling is that they tend to be little things, a little realisation and then a little realisation built on that."

- *Roger Penrose*

Following the clues

We know that intense stress is usually involved at the outset of CFS. We understand the connection between stress hormones, such as adrenaline and cortisol, and bodily dysfunction. However, **if the initial stressor has subsided, then why does the dysfunction continue?**

This was a key question for me. Many things helped me find the answer, but my own experience initially drove me in this direction.

Early in my research, I saw that PECs' ability to deal with stress was diminished. This makes sense. Although we can deal with a great deal of adversity, we will eventually reach a point where we find it difficult to cope. The great work of endocrinologist Hans Selye and the conditions of adrenal insufficiency explain a great deal of this.

As my CFS had progressed, long-time friends had noticed a change in my personality. I had become cranky and highly strung, but that seemed reasonable for someone coping with a debilitating illness. I knew I was not my personality and took no offence when they commented: If I could change in one direction, I knew I could change back again.

However, as I fixed my dysfunctions and my health improved, I noticed that **my reaction to stress was not improving.** As I became more able to cope with daily activities and my sea of emotion and frustration subsided, I expected my short temper, irritability, and overreaction to subside—but they didn't.

As my health continued to improve, my incongruous behaviour was more and more obvious to *me*. (My wife made me emphasise the word *me* here. It had been quite obvious to *her* for a long time.)

I noticed external signs, such as overreacting and raising my voice. I also had internal signs, such as feelings of urgency, anxiety, a need for control, and general stress, often without any reasonable cause. I worried excessively. Whilst I wasn't making up problems or imagining things, I was attuned to any negative or dangerous possibilities, whether for me, my family, my community, my country, or the world in general.

Initially I thought of this as a holdover from my illness. If ordinary activities are difficult, then getting upset can become a habit. But my research showed that my experience was not unique.

I also learned that **PECs tended to have certain personality types.** Earlier, I had dismissed this. Frankly, I was offended by the suggestion that my personality had made me ill, so I understand that others may feel offended too. I am not saying that every PEC develops exactly the same personality changes as I did. But the facts are what they are, and you might see if you notice some of what I describe, or ask those close to you if they have, even if they have not said anything.

I knew that a dysfunction in cortisol regulation could explain CFS. I knew, too, that since I'd been ill my ability to cope with stress and my propensity to create stress had changed. (Remember, stress is a response that comes from a gap, *real or perceived,* between a demand and the ability to meet that demand.) So I had to ask myself:

Since stress hormones seem to play a central role in CFS, and PECs have a diminished ability to deal with stress, was this a key connection?

Could my experience of stress be a sign of a common underlying dysfunction in PECs?

ANS dysfunction

The ANS (autonomic nervous system) operates subconsciously. We don't directly control it. It is the inner part of our brain that ensures that our heart keeps beating, our gut keeps digesting, and we keep breathing, salivating, perspiring, and so on. In regulating some of these functions (such as breathing), it can work together with the conscious mind. (This will be important for treatment.)

As we've seen, the ANS is divided into two main subsystems, the SNS (sympathetic nervous system) and the PNS (parasympathetic nervous system). (There is talk of a third system that uses nitric oxide as a neurotransmitter, but I won't go into that here.)

The SNS controls our stress (fight-or-flight) response and pumps out stress hormones such as adrenaline and cortisol. The PNS counteracts this and promotes maintenance of the body when we are at rest. They work together, in balance.

After much research and thought, it became clear to me that a dysfunction of the ANS would explain the symptoms and conundrums of CFS. This, then, is the hypothesis of this book:

The root cause of CFS is a dysfunction of the ANS that arouses the SNS (to fight-or-flight mode) and the PNS (to rest-and-digest mode) with inappropriate triggers at excessive levels.

It was evidence of the PNS triggering that led me to this conclusion. But the SNS response is more often recognised and discussed because it is usually dominant in the face of stress.

When the SNS is triggered, everything changes, from our heartbeat and blood pressure to our digestion and sleep. **This leads to the constant firing of the hypothalamic–pituitary–adrenal (HPA) axis and overproduction of cortisol. Eventually we end up with a partial** underproduction and overproduction of cortisol at the same time.

Understanding the ANS dysfunction in PECs

Figure 7 shows this central dysfunction or cause of CFS. As you can see in the diagram, a healthy person's ANS is in balance a majority of the time. At some times, the PNS dominates to relax, to digest a heavy meal, or to move towards sleep. At other times, the SNS dominates to cope with any stress experienced.

SNS dominance and the overproduction of stress hormones such as cortisol and adrenaline explain most of the dysfunctions that lead to the symptoms of CFS.

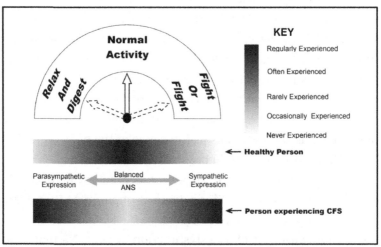

Figure 7: Concept Illustration for Sympathetic and Parasympathetic Imbalance in PECs

However, PNS dominance explains the low cortisol levels of most longer-term PECs as well as the other nervous system dysfunctions. The most obvious of these is Orthostatic Intolerance (OI), which is a common symptom of CFS. Sometimes this is diagnosed as Postural Orthostatic Tachycardia Syndrome (POTS).

OI is essentially the failure of the body to respond properly when a person goes from a lying-down position to an upright one. This is usually felt as light-headedness and heart palpitations or rapid heartbeat as blood pressure drops. It may be the clearest direct expression of the ANS dysfunction. However, other factors are involved, including low blood volume. Low blood volume is caused primarily by chronic underproduction of aldosterone. The production of aldosterone is controlled by the ANS via the HPA axis.

I believe that excessive PNS dominance is a mechanism to shield the body from further SNS dominance. This is closely related to the phenomenon of 'playing dead' or fainting under extreme duress: The PNS activates the vagus nerve and causes a precipitous plunge in blood pressure, leading to a loss in consciousness. **In PECs this phenomenon is more measured, but it likely contributes to the general feeling of malaise and lack of muscle tone during periods of extreme exhaustion.** I have seen direct evidence of this mechanism on my own heart rate under significant exercise stress.

So whilst many of the secondary illnesses—mitochondrial dysfunction, poor liver function, infections, hormone gland depletion, insulin resistance, poor gut function, and so on—need to be addressed, it is this central cause of CFS, the ANS dysfunction which causes excessive SNS and PNS dominance, that needs to be corrected to allow us to return to health.

Let me give you an analogy. Imagine driving a broken car. Instead of responding to varying degrees of pressure on the accelerator and brakes, it acts like a digital switch, fully on or fully off. First you race along at full power, until you run out of gas. You refuel, then at the tiniest touch of the accelerator, it roars off at full speed again. It won't slow down when you want to turn a corner. That vehicle will give you a rough trip. It's only a matter of time before your engine blows up, your tyres melt, or you crash.

Our bodies are similar. If they only have two possibilities—all go or all stop—then our responses can't be healthy.

We'll look at all this a little more closely in the next chapter.

The importance of getting the full picture

You may have heard parts of this hypothesis before and tried treatments without success. This is usually due to the lack of a full understanding of how the ANS interacts with bodily dysfunctions.

Keep reading to the end of this book, as a lot more detail is revealed in the second half.

CHAPTER SUMMARY

- PECs' response to stress is amplified.

- The hypothesis of this book is that the root cause of CFS is a dysfunction of the ANS that arouses the SNS (to fight-or-flight mode) and the PNS (to rest-and-digest mode) with inappropriate triggers at excessive levels.

- Whilst a healthy person's ANS is balanced most of the time, PECs are either in SNS or PNS dominance, with little time spent in a "just right" mode.

- Whilst many of the secondary illnesses—mitochondrial dysfunction, poor liver function, infections, hormone gland depletion, insulin resistance, poor gut function, and so on— need to be addressed, **it is this central cause of CFS, this ANS dysfunction of excessive SNS and PNS dominance, that needs to be corrected to allow us to return to health.**

CHAPTER 13

Putting It All Together

"First, you know, a new theory is attacked as absurd; then it is admitted to be true, but obvious and insignificant; finally it is seen to be so important that its adversaries claim that they themselves discovered it."

- William James

As always, the more answers I found, the more questions I asked. If the ANS dysfunction is the cause of CFS, the next question is;

Why does the ANS dysfunction occur?

The short answer is, the ANS dysfunction occurs as a result of an overwhelming amount of physiological and psychological stress that triggers the SNS. Since the effects of that much stress are unsustainable, the body takes emergency protective measures, including overusing the PNS. Think of it as an emergency circuit breaker.

The long answer is of course more complicated, but our focus here is on practical information to help you recover. (In the video explanation at my website, I touch on additional points.)

We've seen that the HPA axis orders the production of adrenal hormones. If we believe the hypothalamus is firing inappropriately, then we must consider how it is triggered. Let's start with the function of two small, almond-shaped parts of the brain called the amygdalae.

The pathway to trigger the SNS

Figure 8 is a simplified image of how the stress response is produced.

In the lower right corner, we have a stimulus, like seeing a snake or hearing a bang. That data is filtered through the thalamus. **Our bodies then have a choice of three pathways for response.**

The speediest route is via the amygdalae, directly to the hypothalamus. The amygdalae are not discerning; they cannot reason. They help process memories of emotional reactions. This **lightning-fast pathway** is subconscious, so it allows us to respond without thinking. In the face of real danger, the amygdalae provide the fastest possible response. When you hear a loud bang, your HPA axis fires before you even consider what caused it.

The **fast pathway** is similar but detours through the sensory cortex. The brain does a bit more processing to evaluate the stimulus, but it does not carry out a full thought process or bring up other events in our memories. An example of this might be hearing a rattling sound and recognising it as a snake. This then fires the amygdalae.

The **slow pathway** happens in the conscious part of the mind, via the transitional cortex and the hippocampus, where memories are stored. Here you evaluate the stimulus before making a decision. You also program a reaction for the next time you meet the same stimulus.

For example, if you see someone walking towards you in a dark alley, you consider the setting, the time, and the person's walk. When you see that the person is wearing a blue scarf, you remember a newspaper story about a blue-scarf strangler who strikes at this time of the evening, and your HPA axis fires. This reaction feeds back to program your amygdalae. The programming happens regardless of whether you wrestle with the blue-scarf strangler or eventually realise it's just Grandma in a new scarf. The next time you see someone in a dark alley, your stomach might lurch; but it might also lurch the next time you see Grandma. Both have become triggers.

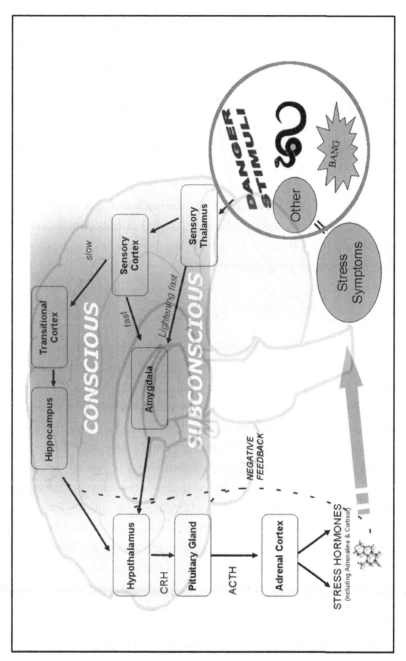

Figure 8: Hypothalamus Trigger

This is how responses are programmed. Anything that causes a strong reaction can thus become a trigger, whether the fear is appropriate (as with the rattle of a snake) or not (as with Grandma or phobias).

With CFS, severe or prolonged stress has turned too many things into triggers, and the body's reactions are too frequent and too strong. **The amygdalae are caught in a feedback loop that keeps them on high alert. They fire the HPA axis over and over at inappropriate triggers.**

This firing causes an excess of adrenal hormones in the body. It eventually leads to reduced overall adrenal output with intermittent excess output. It also leads to the symptoms and secondary dysfunctions that perpetuate the illness.

Triggers

The triggers cause the SNS to produce the cortisol surges that keep PECs up half the night. This depletes cortisol, robbing us of the vitally-needed morning cortisol that gets us out of bed.

I believe that once the ANS dysfunction takes hold, almost anything that is perceived as stress or potential stress can be a trigger. The word *potential* is important here, because it opens a very wide door.

Let me explain. Much psychological stress is caused by imagined events. Simply walking under a bridge does not produce stress. However, if you think the bridge will collapse on you—if, for example, you were recently trapped under the rubble of a collapsed bridge—the perception of danger and impending injury and pain will put you in a highly-stressed state. But your fear does not have to be based on a real experience. You may have heard that bridges have been collapsing lately, or that one bridge collapsed, or that bridges might collapse. Maybe you read a novel where a bridge nearly collapsed.

Any situation that could potentially lead to a stressful event can become a stressful event in its own right. Seeing a bridge or even looking for a bridge can become stressful if this fear is programmed

strongly enough into your nervous system.

If almost anything can become a trigger, PECs have a problem. And one of the most stressful things for a PEC is the illness itself.

I have identified four main triggers of the ANS dysfunction:

1. Physical stress due to bodily dysfunctions (subconscious)
2. Mental and emotional stress about CFS and its symptoms (conscious and subconscious)
3. Mental and emotional stress from the environment (conscious and subconscious)
4. Mental and emotional stress experienced in the past (conscious and subconscious)

I believe that all PECs experience the two first triggers, perhaps the first three if we consider the impact of chronic illness on our lives. Only some of us experience the fourth trigger of past experiences.

ANS kindling

Triggers are not the only problem. When the amygdalae receive danger signals, they also activate a system in the forebrain to release a neurotransmitter called acetylcholine (aCh) throughout the cortex.

The amygdalae also interact with other systems to arouse the brain stem. 'Arousal' refers to the amount of activity in the brain. When we are asleep and not dreaming, arousal is very low. But if we are facing a crisis, our arousal is high; our brain is very active.

Unfortunately, the arousal of the brain feeds back to keep the amygdalae aroused. A loop is formed: The aroused amygdalae arouse the brain, and the aroused brain keeps the amygdalae aroused.

Thanks to the flashbulb-memory effect, memories formed in the brain at such times are stronger. The high level of emotional arousal forms strong neuro associations. Normal and natural concerns about symptoms at this time can transform into powerful triggers of the ANS.

So ANS dysfunction has created a state in the nervous system that allows new triggers to be formed easily. This neurological kindling happens unconsciously or subconsciously.

How CFS self-perpetuates with ANS dysfunction

Figure 9 shows the ANS dysfunction cycle and how CFS self-perpetuates.

As you can see, two cycles directly perpetuate CFS. One is physical triggering of the ANS dysfunction. This is often caused by CFS symptoms and secondary dysfunctions such as hypoglycaemia, infection, dehydration, and toxicity as well as fatigue and pain.

The second is mental and emotional triggers of the ANS dysfunction which are conscious and subconscious. These stressors did not cause CFS, but they perpetuate it. We are not just talking about just feeling low because we are unwell, we are talking about powerful fears associated with CFS!

It's important to realise that these mental or emotional triggers aren't always conscious. So even if we feel little distress and we think we are OK, we may have triggered our ANS simply by searching for symptoms. (Remember the bridge anxiety.) Since much of this process happens subconsciously, becoming aware of it is key. Once we become aware of it, we can stop it.

These are not the only triggers. If they were, all PECs would recover as soon as they went through a period of better health (some PECs do recover this way).

Additional triggers may be mental (such as excessive work hours, feelings of urgency, or difficult and complex tasks) or physical (such as exercise, injury, or infection). One very powerful trigger is emotional stress, which may be caused by life events (such as divorce, loss of a loved one, or being in an abusive relationship).

Once the ANS dysfunction is in place, any trigger can restart the cycle. It also appears that past negative life events that we have not dealt with can also act as triggers, as the unresolved emotions resurface over and over until we find resolution.

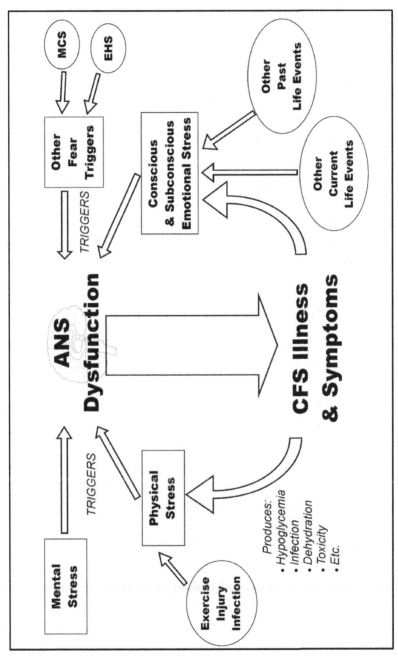

Figure 9: ANS Dysfunction Cycle

PECs may develop other triggers, such as multiple chemical sensitivity (MCS) or electromagnetic hypersensitivity (EHS). **Any event, experience, or exposure that gets neurologically linked as a threat can act as a trigger.** Even things like too much sun exposure, too much noise, or strong vibrations can act as triggers.

However, whilst avoiding a trigger may reduce your symptoms and make you feel better, it is not the same as recovering. It can actually worsen your condition by reinforcing the trigger.

To give you an analogy, if your dog bites every time he hears a ringing sound, it may help to silence your doorbell and telephone, but it's better to retrain your dog.

So for lasting recovery, we must normalise ANS function rather than just avoid the triggers.

The development of CFS in PECs

Figure 10 shows how CFS develops via the ANS dysfunction, and why PECs struggle to recover. It shows three primary cycles and a secondary cycle.

The best way to look at this busy Figure, is to go to the word 'Start' at the top right hand corner.

As you can see, the illness usually begins after a combination of physiological and psychological stressors. This **onset cycle** puts us on the road to CFS. At this time PECs usually experience such things as irritability, tiredness, anxiety, anger, or sadness as well as physical symptoms like feeling run down and tired.

In some cases this onset cycle is started by a physical stressor, like a physical injury, surgery, child birth or excessive exercise, which then leads to psychological stress in connection to that.

In other cases, psychological stress comes first, from a relationship breakdown, exams or some sort of trauma. Then a physical stressor adds more to the burden to tip the system over the edge.

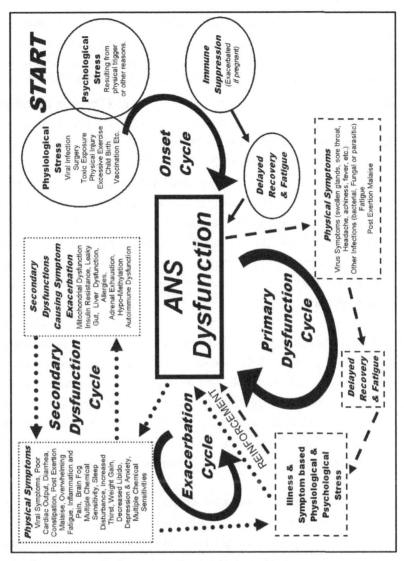

Figure 10: Hypothesis of the Pathogenesis of CFS

Whilst in some cases only one type of stressor (physiological or psychological) occurs, in the vast majority of the time there are stressors of both types. This makes sense given that most physical stress is accompanied by some kind of psychological stress.

Next comes delayed recovery and often fatigue. Recovery is delayed due to the depressed immune system and the drained resources of the body that has been responding to excessive demands.

Now, with high levels of adrenal hormones and a large variety of physical symptoms, the ANS dysfunction occurs. (This is in the middle of the diagram because it is central to CFS.) The ANS becomes SNS dominant and keeps our adrenal hormone levels high. Over time, we start to experience some periods of adrenal insufficiency.

This leads to the **primary dysfunction cycle** of CFS. Typically, we have viral-like symptoms such as swollen glands, sore throat, and headache. We also experience fatigue.

For some people, the start of CFS is clearly marked. Others can't distinguish between the original onset and this cycle but may remember thinking, "I can't believe I am sick again," or "When am I going to get better?"

If this was during or after a period of stress, we were probably busy with important things and didn't take a break to let ourselves recover.

It is only a matter of time before the illness becomes a new source of physiological and psychological stress. A week of sickness can seem like an eternity. But as weeks and then months pass, we begin to worry: "Am I ever going to get well again?" or "What is really wrong with me? This isn't just flu," or "I can't cope."

This stress reinforces the ANS dysfunction. Now we are in a vicious cycle.

Those who recover from CFS within a shorter period of time will usually come out of this cycle within three to six months. However, those who do not recover quickly will experience an **exacerbation cycle** which may lead to further problems. Most of the symptoms continue, and problems like fatigue and digestive dysfunction become worse.

The chronic SNS arousal (the fight-or-flight response) then leads to other problems—a depressed immune system, brain fog or poor cognitive functioning, sleep disturbance, multiple chemical sensitivity, unquenchable thirst, weight gain, decreased libido, anxiety, depression, and so on.

I want to make an important distinction here about depression: If we are depressed at this point, it is a consequence of our illness or alongside it. Depression is *not* the cause of CFS.

All this illness and dysfunction leads to a further cycle. (That's right. Just when we think it can't get worse, it gets worse.) I call this the **secondary dysfunction cycle** as it causes additional conditions. Not everyone with CFS will have all of these conditions. In some cases, these conditions may start first and then lead into or trigger CFS. They can also cause relapses.

These conditions include such things as mitochondrial dysfunction, hypomethylation, insulin resistance, leaky gut, liver dysfunction, and adrenal insufficiency. I believe that the majority of long-term PECs end up with most of these. Other conditions, such as chronic pain, severe allergies and autoimmune dysfunctions, will apply only to some people.

I separate these conditions from the other dysfunctions for this reason: Based on my research in physiology, my own experience, and others' experiences, **I believe that if the ANS dysfunction is corrected, most of these conditions will disappear over time.**

However, PECs who have been ill for a long time may have to address these secondary problems at the same time as they work on the ANS dysfunction. **I believe that ignoring them or treating them incorrectly keeps some long-term PECs from recovering even if they are doing everything else right.** That is because these physical problems can themselves act as triggers or pathways into CFS. They can thus stop PECs from recovering or cause them to relapse.

As you may have gathered, this complex illness can't be easily laid out in a neat diagram. Some dysfunctions may not occur for years after the onset of CFS; or they may start at the onset or even before.

CFS is self-perpetuating. The sickness keeps you sick. Stress causes illness and symptoms, and these in turn cause more stress, which causes more illness.

I want to remind you here that 'stress' doesn't mean just psychological stress. We are also talking about the physiological stress that PECs experience as a result of being ill.

Stress occurs at both conscious and subconscious levels. Conscious stress may come from dealing with the illness and looking out for symptoms; subconscious stress may be due to dysfunctions like low blood sugar or other bodily feedback to which the ANS overreacts.

If all that is not complicated enough, certain aspects of the illness can cause other problems—that is, dysfunction 1 can cause dysfunction 2, which in turn can cause dysfunction 1. Here are some examples:

- Gut dysfunction can lead to nutritional deficiency and toxic exposure, which can lead to hypomethylation and mitochondrial dysfunction, which in turn can lead to gut dysfunction.
- Oxidative stress can lead to hypomethylation, which can lead to reduced glutathione production, which can lead to oxidative stress.
- Mitochondrial dysfunction can lead to reduced cardiac output, which can lead to reduced blood supply, which can lead to mitochondrial dysfunction.

I could go on, but let me try to simplify all of this.

I believe that the cause of CFS is the ANS dysfunction, which produces inappropriate stress responses to a variety of triggers. These responses in turn perpetuate CFS symptoms. Along with this, a variety of secondary illnesses develop and perpetuate. These also feed back to trigger the ANS dysfunction as well as other bodily dysfunctions.

CFS therefore perpetuates itself until all cycles are interrupted and the dysfunctions are corrected.

Perhaps the easiest way to explain how this hypothesis works is by using an imaginary PEC. Let's call her Mary.

Mary: The hypothesis in action

Like the average person these days, Mary starts off in a state of suboptimal health.

Her diet is high in stimulants—coffee, cola, tea, energy drinks—and sugars. By 'sugars', I mean not just sweets but also carbohydrates, like bread, which Mary has every day. She has regular, sizeable servings of pasta, potatoes, and rice, with plenty of beans, peas, lentils, chickpeas, and similar products like hummus and mashes. She drinks high-sugar drinks like sodas and juice. (That's right, orange and apple juice have the same sugar content as soft drinks like cola. Many juices are even higher, up to fifty percent higher.)

All this sugar over a period of years has led to a bit of insulin resistance in Mary, but she's not aware of it because it's too little to show up clinically or cause noticeable problems.

Mary eats what she feels is a 'reasonable' amount of fresh fruit and vegetables, but she has a poor vitamin and mineral intake given the reduced nutritional content of foods grown with modern farming techniques. The vegetables that she does eat are usually cooked and leached of their nutrients. However, this has not caused her any real bother yet either. Remember, the body is amazing at compensating.

But things change when life hits an inevitable speed bump. Perhaps her boss makes extra demands on her, her husband gets seriously ill, or she loses a family member. Maybe she's going through a divorce or she decides to break the world record for successive marathons. If Mary is like most people, it's usually a couple of things at once. What we do know is that it's huge, maybe more stress than ever before in her life.

But Mary has a certain type of personality. She is tougher than the average person. She doesn't give up easily, she fights on, she can handle it! Mary carries on under this high stress level for so long, it almost becomes a new normal. She thinks she's coping well, but her friends see she is wound up like a spring.

Then something else happens, something physical. She gets her wisdom teeth out, or maybe catches up on all her vaccinations at once for her big trip overseas, or maybe she just gets the flu from hell. Let's assume it's the flu.

Because her cortisol levels have been high for some time, Mary's immune system is depressed. She struggles to get over this flu. Since Mary is a fighter, she takes flu pills and keeps going to work, looking after her family, and doing everything else she needs to do.

The flu gets worse. Now she is too sick to get out of bed, with headaches, a sore throat, fever, and severe lethargy. Her herpes virus flares up, too. She eventually gets well enough to be back at work. But she's not fully well, so her symptoms get worse again.

Suddenly, besides being stressed out and highly strung, she starts to worry: Should she take it easy? Does she have something worse than the flu? Her doctor says it's just post-viral fatigue and she'll get over it shortly. He notes that she seems distressed and offers to prescribe something for depression.

Mary tries to take it easy, but she has too much to do.

She scans her body for symptoms, in case she needs to slow down, because she can't afford to end up back in bed. Her cortisol levels are not getting any lower. In fact, they are higher, since being sick gives her a new set of worries. When she notices symptoms or feels worse, she tenses up: Flu doesn't normally last for sixteen weeks!

What Mary doesn't realise is that her amygdalae have started to experience neurological kindling. They now react to *any* stressors, physical or mental. Even thinking about being unwell contributes to her problem. The flashbulb-memory effect ensures that she will have a strong reaction to those thoughts. They trigger her fight-or-flight response, which leads to the release of more cortisol. The chronically high levels of cortisol then make her symptoms worse—and the longer she is unwell, the more symptoms and problems she accumulates.

When the amygdalae react to these 'dangers', they also signal to her brain to keep it aroused. Unfortunately, this arousal feeds back to keep her amygdalae aroused, forming another loop. Since these loops are unconscious or subconscious, Mary is not even aware of them.

Mary's thoughts about being unwell get darker. She thinks about all the things she has missed out on in the last month and what will happen if she stays sick. These conscious thoughts further arouse her amygdalae and become triggers, too.

Now Mary's neuro-endocrine system is out of control. Its feedback cycle reinforces its reactions. The amygdalae see physical symptoms as danger and react, even when Mary isn't conscious of them. Even conscious thoughts that were previously not a problem now trigger a strong response from her ANS.

Mary has just started the chronic part of her syndrome. The longer it goes on, the bigger impact it will have on Mary's body, and the more entrenched her condition becomes.

Over time, secondary problems develop. Her depressed glutathione levels cause a problem with her methylation, interfering with her liver's ability to detoxify her body. This, along with her inability to absorb essential amino acids, throws her neurotransmitters out of balance. Her serotonin and melatonin levels drop. More and more problems accumulate. More and more symptoms show up.

For a brief while, she begins to feel better. Unfortunately, this is because her adrenals glands are now producing less cortisol. They are trying to balance her system and return her body to homeostasis. And even though her cortisol levels have temporarily dropped, new problems have been created.

Mary's hippocampus has shrunk due to the high cortisol levels. She can't see it, but she notices she's begun to have memory problems.

Unluckily for Mary, the hippocampus is also responsible for down-regulating and counteracting the signals from the amygdalae to the HPA axis. Now her amygdalae are totally out of control.

She hasn't noticed these effects, but her friends have. Mary is a little jumpier, a little more down, a little more worried about everything around her. Her friends put it down to the stress of not being well.

But then Mary starts to act strange. She is experiencing severe pain, yet doctors can't find a source for it. She jumps and cries out at even light pressure on certain tender points, and at times she struggles even with the touch of her blouse on her skin. Mary eventually gets diagnosed with fibromyalgia.

And as the effects of an overactive SNS continue to take their toll on Mary's body, her cortisol levels whilst still spiking, are starting to become severely low. Her adrenals that regulate her minerals are causing her to lose precious minerals like magnesium, sodium and potassium. Even worse, her mineral levels and mineral ratios are so out of balance, that she starts to develop muscle spasms and eventually experiences irregular heart-beats.

When she experiences a stressor, physical or mental, she notices how her body and brain suddenly shuts down, like a switch. She notices how she goes from one moment to the next, suddenly feeling completely foggy, completely listless, like someone pulled out the plug. What Mary doesn't realise is that her ANS is now expressing the rest and digest response (PNS), or more accurately, an extreme version called the 'play dead' reflex.

Mary feels faint when she stands up, but it's just another symptom. But when she faints one day, she falls and hits her head and ends up in hospital. The doctors do a range of new tests and ask her about her palpitations. They diagnose Mary with Postural Orthostatic Tachycardia Syndrome (POTS).

Then she claims that chemicals are making her sick. Her sense of smell is connected to parts of her amygdalae, which are on high alert, looking for and reacting to further potential dangers. The moment she smells perfumes or petrochemical compounds she flees. Mary is experiencing Multiple Chemical Sensitivities (MCS).

Eventually, she asks her friends to switch off their mobile phones when they visit. Mary is experiencing Electromagnetic Hypersensitivity (EHS).

Her friends wonder if it is all in her head. Maybe Mary is depressed. Maybe she is a hypochondriac.

Little do they realise that the areas in the brain associated with pain processing have lit up like a Christmas tree and that Mary's pain is real and severe.

Little do they realise that her olfactory bulb and olfactory cortex are directly connected to the cortical nucleus of her Amygdalae which are on high alert looking out for any further potential dangers. Whilst a whiff of perfume or petrol doesn't carry much toxic load, her amygdalae's response to it creates consequences that are severe and real.

Little do they realise that Mary has CFS.

CHAPTER SUMMARY

- This book proposes that the ANS dysfunction occurs because of an overwhelming amount of physical and psychological stress. The body's attempt to cope with this unsustainable stress and return to homeostasis leads to neurological kindling, in which the ANS starts to react inappropriately to stressors.

- The amygdalae are the fastest pathway to activating the SNS (the fight-or-flight response). This pathway is meant to be used in the face of real danger. The amygdalae operate largely subconsciously; they are not discerning and cannot reason.

- According to this book's hypothesis, PECs' amygdalae fire the HPA axis at inappropriate triggers, including the following:

  - Physical stress due to bodily dysfunctions
  - Mental or emotional stress about CFS and its symptoms
  - Mental or emotional stress from the environment
  - Mental or emotional stress experienced in the past

- This hypothesis of CFS proposes three main cycles plus a secondary illness cycle.

  - The **onset cycle** starts with physiological and psychological stress leading to immune suppression and a delayed recovery.

  - Then the **ANS dysfunction** occurs. This is the central cause of CFS.

  - Next, the **primary dysfunction cycle** creates a variety of symptoms including fatigue, infections, and immune system symptoms such as swollen glands.

  - The **exacerbation cycle** includes the problems of the primary cycle as well inflammation, widespread pain, brain fog, poor cognitive functioning, sleep disturbance, weight gain, decreased libido, depression, and anxiety.

  - During the **secondary dysfunction cycle,** dysfunctions are created that can perpetuate in their own right and that may need to be addressed separately. These may also act as triggers for the start of CFS or for a relapse.

continued

- CFS does not fit neatly into a diagram, as the dynamics are complicated.
- CFS perpetuates CFS. Whilst the primary problem is the ANS dysfunction, the secondary cycles of CFS may also need to be interrupted to overcome long-term CFS.

Part Three:
THE PATH TO RECOVERY

IMPORTANT WARNING:

As stated in the front of this book, this book is not intended to replace your physician and is not a substitute for medical diagnosis, advice, or treatment. Please consult your doctor first, before you embark on any of the processes or treatments described in this book and before you discontinue any medications. I recommend that all readers also consult with their medical doctor before starting any supplements, among other reasons to ensure that there is no incompatibility with any medication.

If you have not been formally diagnosed by a medical doctor with CFS or one of its variants, I recommend that you seek to clarify the nature of your condition before proceeding with any treatments described in this book. CFS diagnosis is usually made after a process of elimination of other diseases. It is important to ensure that you are not suffering from some other disease that should be treated by your doctor. This step is ABSOLUTELY CRITICAL and you must take part in a diligent process of elimination BEFORE trying to treat CFS.

CHAPTER 14

Treatments 'with' or 'to' your body?

"Control what you can control. Don't lose sleep worrying about things that you don't have control over because, at the end of the day, you still won't have any control over them."

— Cam Newton

A PEC's frustrating chat:

The doctor/naturopath:	The Patient:
"You've got spastic colon."	*"Aha"*
"You have Candida in your gut."	*"Aha"*
"You've got irritable bowel syndrome."	
	"Yes, this is irritating me!"
"You have parasites in your gut."	
"You have leaky gut."	
	"I tell you what I have; I have had a gut full!"
"You have toxic overload."	
"You have a fatty liver."	
"You have hepatitis."	
"You have alcohol intolerance."	

"You have a chemical intolerance."

"I sure am feeling intolerant now!"

"You have hypoglycaemia."

"You have insulin resistance."

"What am I resisting?"

"You have low DHEA."

"You have adrenal insufficiency."

"You have low cortisol hormone."

"You have low Aldosterone hormone."

"You have low thyroid hormone."

"You have low testosterone hormone."

"Are you saying that I am hormonal?"

"Yes, you have low serotonin."

"You have low melatonin."

"Low melatonin? But I'm getting sleepy right now."

"You have low digestive enzymes."

"You have a mineral imbalance."

"You have inflammation."

"You have cardiac arrhythmia."

"You have a viral infection."

"You have a bacterial infection."

"You have a fungal infection."

"You have autoimmune disorders."

"ALRIGHT, ALRIGHT, I get it. I am sick."

"Are you feeling down? – It's probably depression."

"You forgot something."

"I am not finished – I am only half way."

"I have a headache."

"I don't see any reason for a headache.......You have hypochondria."

"You have ...

CFS is no laughing matter, but hopefully you relate to the frustration of this little conversation with at least a bit of a smile. Long ago I heard these words and they resonated so strongly with me that I never forgot them:

> *"Humour is the human antidote to suffering."*
>
> *- Deepak Chopra*

This little conversation was not just to try to bring a little smile to your face, but to show the huge scope of trying to fix all the problems people endure with this syndrome.

So first of all, we must consider our approach to recovery!

We can spend years trying to fix the individual things that are wrong without ever dealing with the root cause. Yes, PECs do experience a lot of dysfunctions. But trying so many treatments is both emotionally and financially exhausting. So I recommend a different approach.

I believe that understanding CFS and addressing concerns in the right order is critical. But, most importantly, we should also focus on treating the root cause: the ANS dysfunction.

The premise

"Mix salt and sand, and it shall puzzle the wisest of men, with his mere natural appliances, to separate all the grains of sand from all the grains of salt; but a shower of rain will effect the same object in ten minutes."

Thomas Henry Huxley

I consider one premise to be very important for recovery from CFS:

"The human body is an amazingly complex system that is perfectly designed to function well and to restore itself to a healthy state."

What does this mean? It means that perhaps we shouldn't interfere too much with our biochemistry.

PECs and their health practitioners often try to fix the many dysfunctions of CFS. Whist many of these do need restoring, others may exist for a good reason. Perhaps 'fixing' them is not the best idea.

Doctors usually prescribe medication, which can offer some relief from symptoms but does not necessarily solve the underlying problem. On the other hand, naturopaths focus more on building health, but they may use supplements to stimulate functions, perhaps without necessarily understanding the full consequences.

For example, treating dysfunctions such as adrenal insufficiency or hypomethylation may have negative consequences.

Let me explain what I mean. If your hyperaroused ANS is causing your HPA axis to release excessive adrenal hormones, is adrenal insufficiency such a bad thing? Sure, it makes you feel terrible and causes so many symptoms that whole books have been written about it. But—to go back to the broken-car analogy—do we really want a fully-fueled engine powering this dysfunction?

Also, correcting under-methylation will help restore your ability to produce glutathione for detoxification, but can your liver cope with this? Improving methylation may also help you to make aCh, but do you really want more aCh, given its role in brain arousal? What will happen to your dopamine levels if you suddenly become better at breaking this hormone down?

I am not saying that we should live with our dysfunctions, but we need to consider how aggressively to treat them. The body is a delicate balancing act. Every process and hormone has an impact and a counterbalancing process and hormone. Changes in one function may have negative impacts on another. One physicist put it this way:

> *"To every action there is always an equal and opposite reaction"*
> *(Translated from the original Latin text)*
>
> Sir Isaac Newton

If we change how a hormone is made, have we changed how it is metabolised? If not, it will affect overall hormone levels, which we may not want. If we affect one process, what happens to the counterbalancing process? How will that affect the body?

Because of the complexity of the human body and the wisdom of its design, I suggest a conservative, supportive approach rather than an aggressive one. The body knows how to function perfectly. We must always be careful that interventions do not have negative impacts.

The body should lead its own recovery so that it can rebalance its functions. I believe that more aggressive intervention should be considered only in rare cases, where time and normalisation of the ANS have not returned a PEC to health.

However, that doesn't mean that we should do nothing. Some intervention should be considered immediately, to ease symptoms and pave the road to recovery. Treating dysfunctions, providing the right nutrients through diet and supplements, and creating the right environment for healing are essential.

Pharmaceutical assistance

The general medical community has been trained to heal primarily with pharmaceuticals. However, drugs place a toxic burden on the body, and most PECs (particularly those with MCS) already struggle to cope with their toxic load. In my opinion, many PECs are held back from recovery by taking too many drugs, because they add to the burden on an already malfunctioning system.

Drugs can also have many side effects, some of them severe. (Remember the 'equal and opposite reaction'.)

Drugs often treat symptoms rather than fixing underlying problems. **Covering up symptoms is not the same as restoring health.** You don't clean a room by covering the mess with a sheet.

Even more important, we don't want to lose touch with what's going on in our bodies. Symptoms are signs along the road to good health. If we mask our symptoms, how do we know what is still wrong?

Yes, we want to get rid of them eventually, but while we still have them, we don't want to ignore them or cover them up.

Still, I don't suggest taking an extreme position against drugs. They can help if they are used conservatively and wisely. **Stopping medication or hormone therapy suddenly or without the supervision and advice of a doctor is a very bad idea and potentially dangerous.** When you stop using drugs abruptly, they can have rebound effects that amplify dysfunctions. Speak to your doctor, and explore options to reduce your drug intake if it is appropriate.

Keeping a balanced view is also important. Some naturopaths will tell you that all drugs are bad and warn you to stay away from them. But for years, I suffered periods of excruciating pain. It would take days or weeks to pass and often left me unable to get out of bed or function. Over time, the ability to cope with pain diminishes. I had gone from taking no pain medication to swallowing pain killers like candy with little or no effect. (This was not kind to my liver.) One day, a doctor said that the pain was due to inflammation and gave me a drug that I took once. The next day I was astounded to wake up to find that the pain was gone.

Now, don't get me wrong, that drug didn't always work and it was far from a lasting solution. And such drugs have negative side-effects, so I wouldn't have wanted to take them all the time. I needed to fix the underlying problem. But clearly, a treatment option such as this can have real value in the short term. It can help you start your recovery.

Whilst I realise that many doctors will not agree with me, I am also concerned about hormone therapy. Medical science has a reasonable understanding of hormone regulation, but I do not believe we have a full understanding. Taking hormones without understanding the full, long-term impact is clearly not without risks.

For example, some doctors prescribe hydrocortisone for adrenal insufficiency. (I'll discuss this in more detail later.) In my opinion, this may further inhibit hormone production via feedback loops. The doctor may refer to studies showing that low-level supplementation does not have this impact, but these studies were not done specifically on PECs with a malfunctioning HPA axis. If you take in a 'normal' amount of hormone, then have an extreme surge from time to time, the body can down-regulate the hormone further before too much damage is done.

My view is, that it is prudent to be very careful about all kinds of hormone therapy. In some instances, it may be appropriate (like with some hormone precursors). You will need to be guided by your doctor, but my advice is always to **seek a qualified second opinion from a holistic doctor before making a final decision.**

Also discuss in some detail your doctor's experience with the type of treatment and what longer-term success his patients have had with that approach. **Perhaps most importantly, discuss the impact of ceasing such a therapy.**

CHAPTER SUMMARY

- Try to develop a more light-hearted approach to your CFS challenge.

- The natural state of the body is to be healthy. The body knows best. Some dysfunctions have an unknown benefit or reason for existing that may not be apparent.

- A balanced, conservative approach is desirable as opposed to extreme drug-intensive or drug-aversive viewpoints.

- Too much medication can add to the toxic burden in PECs.

- **Never stop or start medication, hormone therapy, or powerful nutrition or supplement treatments without the supervision and advice of a medical doctor.**

- **Always seek a qualified second opinion regarding drug and hormone therapies.**

CHAPTER 15

The Master Plan

"A good battle plan that you act on today can be better than a perfect one tomorrow."

- General George S Patton

The key word in the above quote is 'good'. Rushing into a bad plan will spell disaster. However, waiting until you have worked out a perfect process may mean never getting started. The best solution, once again, is a balanced approach.

A skilled and experienced holistic or integrative doctor will treat the different dysfunctions of CFS in a specific order, based on one part science, one part experience, and one part intuition. I won't detail this order here. I suggest that you don't become absorbed in such details or continue endlessly researching naturopathic or integrative medicine. Instead, be the macro-manager—the CEO—of your recovery, and choose the right practitioners to guide you.

Remember: **The human body is an amazingly complex system that is perfectly designed to function well and restore itself to a healthy state.** Have some faith in your body's ability to heal itself once the underlying problems are fixed.

Some approaches that only correct the stress response can have reasonable success with PECs. As the body begins to function normally, a lot of problems resolve themselves on their own. However, this may not work with PECs who have been ill for a long time or who have severe and multiple secondary dysfunctions. In these cases, I think a more comprehensive approach makes much more sense.

Also, we need to approach a recovery plan at an appropriate pace, allowing for differences in individual circumstances. Rushing the process can cause problems and setbacks. **It is important to listen to your body.** Suggesting that you don't recover too quickly may sound absurd, but please consider this point carefully, because the body maintains a delicate balance. Fixing one thing without fixing all the counterbalances can produce negative results.

Broadly speaking, I believe that PECs should think of recovery as having four stages. I will outline the steps here and then go into more detail in subsequent sections.

Stage 1: Get started and put out the fires

We cannot do everything in a day. Recovery usually takes time and effort. Where do we start?

If the underlying cause of CFS is the ANS dysfunction, it makes sense to focus on resetting your ANS.

However, for many PECs, certain symptoms may be so extreme that it is difficult to do much. These may include severe fatigue, pain and inflammation, stiffness, and flulike and intestinal symptoms. Some simple things will likely give you significant relief in a short period of time. (Of course, these should be done under the guidance and supervision of your doctor and naturopath.)

Let's start with an action list.

1. Build your team: Find a holistic doctor you feel comfortable with who has some experience with CFS. This may be worth a little effort. If you are already working with a doctor who is not trained in orthomolecular medicine (healing using nutrition and supplements), try to find a naturopath to work with as well. Communication between the two is important. If they are in conflict, you may have to replace one or both or find a holistic doctor.

2. Find a person to support you in your recovery. Your partner or immediate family may be suffering from support burnout. They may have heard enough about this challenge of yours; some may see your situation as hopeless. A person with a fresh perspective who has faith in your recovery can be very valuable, in encouraging you and reminding you of your overall progress. It is a good idea for them to read this book so they can remind you of what you need to do to stay on track.

3. Read the section in this book on ANS normalisation and pain desensitisation and start working on that.

4. Normalise your mineral balance. Your medical advisers will likely run blood and hair mineral analyses, but you can be pretty sure that you lack magnesium, particularly if you feel stiff in the morning. This is my first recommendation for anyone with CFS. I believe that significant amounts (around 300–500 mg per day) are likely to have an impact within as little as a month or two. Those suffering from adrenal insufficiency will likely have low sodium, leading to salt cravings. Adding more salt to your diet will also reduce orthostatic intolerance symptoms (where standing up causes dizziness). The quality of the salt is important. It is also important to monitor sodium levels, as ongoing excessive salt consumption can be harmful.

5. IMPORTANT: If you have hypertension (high blood pressure), increasing salt intake could be dangerous. In this case, do not use this strategy and seek medical advice.

6. Discuss options for pain management with your doctor. There are no magic solutions for pain, but getting temporary relief or reducing pain levels can help you function better and maintain your recovery efforts. Most medications have side effects, and some can cause problems when you stop using them. I suggest using them

sparingly, if possible, because drugs can add to your toxic burden, especially if you are taking other medications.

7. Change your diet. Certain problems can be significantly reduced or eliminated by fine-tuning your diet, including hypoglycaemia, candida, insulin resistance, cellular nutritional deficit, adrenal insufficiency, hormone production problems, and irritable bowel syndrome. Read the section on diet, and get advice tailored to your challenges from your naturopath or holistic doctor.

8. Get nutritional support. Some PECs have a lot of dysfunctions, so your doctor or naturopath may want to prescribe every supplement they carry. Such an approach won't 'fix' you, and in some cases I have seen an aggressive approach make people worse. However, in addition to magnesium, you should at least take the major building blocks for cellular energy production, such as the B vitamins and a quality vitamin C.

Stage 2: Persist and build your recovery

This stage will occur from four to twelve weeks into your recovery, depending on your circumstances and efforts. You will likely no longer be bedridden with flu-like symptoms and you will have some measure of energy. Whilst you may not be able to do major exercise, you can get through the day reasonably well at least some of the time. This is the time to redouble your efforts and forge ahead with these steps.

1. Continue your ANS normalisation and pain desensitisation program.

2. Make significant changes to your diet. Focus on making any major changes needed in your diet, as outlined in this book.

3. Continue with nutritional support. In addition to magnesium and other energy-production supplements, take supplements for any trace minerals if tests indicate that this is necessary.

Rebuild healthy gut flora. Take supplements for other challenges as needed.

4. Read the section in this book on exercise. Exercise is the undoing of many PECs, but the right exercise can be beneficial. Start exercising as soon as you feel well enough.

5. Get enough good quality sleep. Read the section in this book on lifestyle and attitude and develop good sleep habits. Consider nutritional support. As your neurotransmitter balances and functions improve, your sleep will improve.

Stage 3: Deal with any remaining dysfunctions

It can be difficult to know when to deal with remaining dysfunctions such as adrenal insufficiency or under-methylation. In my opinion, the most important thing is to restore your ability to cope with mental stress.

Once the ANS is no longer in overdrive, you can raise your health to the next level. But addressing these dysfunctions just because you are feeling generally well may spell disaster. **You should make sure that you have stopped suffering adrenal surges.**

When you have worked on normalising your ANS for some time, you will probably notice when you have surges. If you don't notice, you will get clues like a sudden change in bowel habit, burning or heat on your upper chest and the back of your neck, hot flashes, sweating, or even a return to sleeplessness or sudden waking in the middle of the night. When these happen, don't worry about them. **It is important to stay calm. Setbacks are a natural part of many recoveries.** Think of them as a welcome opportunity to change your neuro-associations and interrupt the pattern. (You can read more about this in the ANS normalisation section.)

Your focus should be on the following:

1. Continue with the ANS normalisation and pain desensitisation program.

2. Maintain a healthy and supportive diet. Whilst you may relax your diet a little, it is important not to abandon it.

3. Maintain nutritional support. Keep taking some magnesium and essential B vitamins, as directed by your health professional.

4. Keep an eye on your lifestyle and attitude. Keep following the guidelines for a balanced lifestyle and excellent sleeping habits.

5. Address any final disorders such as adrenal insufficiency or under-methylation.

Just a note: For some PECs, this may be a period of reasonable health, but it may still be very frustrating because it can take a little while to get to the point where the body's systems finally balance and our recovery becomes robust. So persist, and remember the words of a former British Prime Minister:

> *"...never give in, never give in, never, never, never, never—in nothing, great or small, large or petty—never give in except to convictions of honour and good sense."*
>
> *Winston Churchill, Oct 29, 1941.*

Sometimes you may feel caught in a version of the-chicken-and-the-egg question: Which comes first, the full restoration of health or the full correction of the ANS dysfunction?

That is, if you continue to look for and treat symptoms, you will likely perpetuate the ANS dysfunction that is causing the symptoms. But if you don't treat your stubborn secondary dysfunctions, how will you reduce them enough to stop triggering the ANS dysfunction? I cover this question in the section entitled; ANS Normalisation: The Chicken or the Egg Conundrum.

Stage 4: Live well and stay well

How long will it take to recover? I can't give you a definite answer, because it depends largely on the individual—not only on their specific physical state, **but also on their personal circumstances and the degree to which they stay the course.**

The treatment for CFS isn't just taking a pill. Recovery doesn't result from a silver bullet cure, it results from a process that is somewhat tailored to the individual and requires follow-through.

Unfortunately, many people feel better and then stop doing all the things they need to. **They don't push on until they are fully well.**

It is up to you whether you do what needs to be done. Only you can change your thought patterns, get help to heal your gut, address childhood trauma, or leave an abusive relationship. Only you can improve your diet, create a healing environment, and do the mental exercises required.

Personal responsibility is a double-edged sword. It means that you have the power to change your life for the better (although you may not believe that until you have made significant progress). It also means you have nobody else to blame. Even if you have a good reason for not doing something, it won't change the outcome.

On the other hand, you need to be kind and gentle with yourself. Self-blame will likely derail your progress. When you are diminished by a chronic illness, it's normal not to follow your plans as well as you would like to. What matters most is that you persist.

Having said that, I will give you an estimate of how long recovery takes, based on anecdotal evidence and my own opinion.

I define recovery as regaining 90-100% or more of your normal health. Depending on your individual issues, how long you have had CFS, and how diligently you follow the program, recovery is likely to take between three and twenty-four months. You may feel recovered within twelve months and sometimes in as little as six months. My expectation is that most people will see a significant improvement (50% to 70%) within six months, but sometimes in as little as three.

If you have been unwell for only three to six months, recovery will likely be quicker. But in my opinion, PECs who suffer significant symptoms for longer than two years or who are taking a large number of medications may take longer to recover even once the ANS dysfunction is corrected. This is because it takes time to wean yourself off these drugs, plus time for your liver to recover, your adrenals and other glands to rebuild, and your body to detoxify. And besides restoring your health, you will also need to restore your muscle tone and endurance.

Once you have recovered 85% or more of your health, it is important to continue to maintain and strengthen it and aim for full recovery. It's my belief that some people who have experienced CFS, may have developed a predisposition to it. This is because the nervous system doesn't forget. Since its reaction is a protective mechanism (to slow you down before you damage yourself with excessive stress), it is likely always to remember this protective strategy.

Don't let that discourage you. It does not mean that you will have a major relapse. **But it does mean that you cannot abuse your body or mind** in the way you may have done before you got ill. So if you learn the lessons of this experience, then you may be less likely to get this illness again compared to people who never learned these lessons.

Yes, you can again be fully active, work full time, exercise, eat a normal diet, and even overindulge in food and drink from time to time. But you may not want to seek a job as a combat soldier, an emergency room physician, or an air traffic controller, or work in any other extremely stressful environment whilst surviving on a diet of Twinkies and watermelon.

Instead, it is critical that you do the following:

1. **Get on with your life and forget about CFS.** Excessive attention to the illness will not help you. Stop looking for bad health, and find something else to focus on, such as a lifelong aspiration, a hobby, or whatever motivates you.

2. **Maintain a reasonable diet.** You don't have to spend the rest of your days eating like Mr. or Ms. Olympia, but make sure that

any splurges are dwarfed by good eating habits and that you normally follow the guidelines for the recovery diet.

3. **Maintain nutritional support.** Few people get the vital minerals that they need. It makes sense to take a few key supplements that are difficult to get from food in the right doses. You may want to take a good quality multivitamin, a vitamin B complex and/or a vitamin B12 supplement (especially if you don't eat much meat), and of course a little magnesium.

4. **Maintain a reasonable lifestyle.** Imagine hearing this from someone who has recovered from CFS; "I worked all night and never stopped to eat anything. It was crazy for three or four days. It was nonstop, and I got hardly any sleep. Now I am sick again. I can't believe it. There is obviously something wrong with me, since I keep getting CFS." Yes, there is something wrong: The person is acting foolishly and self-sabotaging. They need to reconsider their priorities.

5. **Build your health and strength.** Once you feel well again, build your health further. (I discuss exercise in detail in a coming section.) As long as you keep to the guidelines, I believe that you can build up excellent cardiovascular and muscular conditioning with good flexibility. Think of it as insurance. Why settle for being as healthy as everyone else? Why not be healthier? Do proceed slowly and gently. Most PECs won't become professional athletes, although I know of several who have become Olympic or world-class competitors. **I believe that PECs can not only recover but become healthier and stronger than the average person,** even if that seems an impossible stretch right now.

Finding skilled help

If you have been unwell with CFS for a number of years, chances are that you have seen many doctors. So you may be reluctant to go off to see another one. In fact, nearly all the PECs who reviewed my book early on objected to this advice, sometimes very strongly.

I understand this. It is a perfectly reasonable objection. However, even if your previous doctors were not very understanding, this does not mean that you cannot find a doctor who can help you. More and more doctors these days understand a little about CFS and are learning about holistic or integrative medicine. You can benefit greatly from their advice and guidance. If you do not already have this important help on your side, I encourage you to renew your search for it.

If your doctor doesn't know much about orthomolecular medicine, then you will need a skilled naturopath.

Finding the right help is not always easy. However, the rewards are worth the effort. I know that if you dedicate yourself to finding such a person, you will find them. Use everything at your disposal. Here are some ideas of how to go about it:

- Browse the Internet with multiple search terms such as "holistic doctor" +"integrative medicine" + "Chronic Fatigue Syndrome" (or + "Fibromyalgia") + your location.
- Visit chat rooms for PECs. Don't get too drawn into any negativity; use it to find a doctor and/or naturopath.
- Visit a CFS support group in your area. Discussions with other PECs will quickly give you an idea of who is good and who is less helpful.
- Search for doctors that are trained in the Yasko protocol or are part of the Walsh Institute. They will be able to help you restore nutritional balance in your body. If they say they can't help PECs, then just ask them if they are happy to help you normalise your gut function, deal with allergies, and provide dietary advice.

- If none of these things work for you, you might try this. Contact laboratories in your area and ask which doctors order certain tests. You might find out what medical doctors order hair or mineral analyses, saliva cortisol levels, or even bowel flora analyses. Another way is to go into supplement stores and ask the staff if they know of any doctors who recommend supplements or who specialise in CFS. Be resourceful.

CHAPTER SUMMARY

- Don't wait for the perfect recovery plan, but consider your actions and decisions carefully.

- Have some faith in your body's ability to heal itself once the underlying problems are fixed.

- Consider a more comprehensive approach, which is likely to get faster results than just focusing on correcting the ANS dysfunction.

- Adjust the focus of your treatment as you go through the stages of your recovery.

- Work on all aspects of your recovery, including the following:
  - Building a team to support and advise you
  - Normalising your ANS function
  - Normalising pain perception
  - Normalising your mineral balance
  - Evaluating your medical treatment
  - Changing your diet
  - Supplement to overcome nutritional deficiencies;

- Once you have recovered 85% or more of your health, continue to maintain and strengthen it. Don't settle for good health; strive for excellent health.

CHAPTER 16

ANS Normalisation

"Success is in the details."

- Zig Ziglar

In essence, the ANS dysfunction is an inappropriate and ongoing stress response to a variety of triggers. How do we disrupt it?

You may be amazed at how far you have already come, just by realising that this dysfunction is central.

Let me recap the four main triggers of the ANS dysfunction, before we review each in detail:

1. **Physical stress due to bodily dysfunctions (subconscious)**
2. **Mental and emotional stress about CFS and its symptoms (conscious and subconscious)**
3. **Mental and emotional stress from the environment (conscious and subconscious)**
4. **Mental and emotional stress experienced in the past (conscious and subconscious)**

1. Physical stress due to bodily dysfunctions (subconscious)

This is no surprise to anyone experiencing CFS. When you overexert yourself, you will often experience flare-ups. However, it isn't just about physical exertion; it is about understanding the physiological triggers of the ANS dysfunction.

These include the following:

- Hypoglycaemic episodes caused by poor blood sugar regulation
- Excessive oxidative damage due to poor detoxification and toxic sources such as leaky gut
- Abnormal hormone levels
- Dehydration.

You remove these stresses primarily by returning to good health. However, lifestyle choices can drastically reduce them in the meantime. Diet, hydration, sleep, and exercise are critical, especially in the early stages. See the sections of this book on these topics, and take action in these areas.

As you work on the other triggers of the ANS dysfunction, you will normalise the ANS stress response. The stress from bodily dysfunctions should then also decrease, because, as your ANS becomes less reactive, you will create fewer symptoms or physical dysfunctions. For example, as your body stops overreacting to low blood sugar, it will be less likely to have excessive cortisol, adrenalin, and insulin responses.

2. Mental and emotional stress about CFS and its symptoms (conscious and subconscious)

Until I learned what was at the heart of this illness and how the nervous system works, discussions of mental stress and emotions probably would have offended me. It would have been a bit like suggesting that PECs are hypochondriacs or worry-warts.

However, once you understand how the ANS works and how neurological kindling can create a range of triggers—including to generally benign things like smells, EM radiation, flashing lights, or even sounds—it becomes clear that even our mental processes can affect our well-being.

This should be no surprise. Most PECs know that when they experience periods of mental stress, they feel worse. And what could be more stressful than the illness itself?

Conscious stress and subconscious stress are intimately connected. Research shows that the actions and thoughts of the conscious mind can program or influence the subconscious mind.

For example, if you have a phobia about mice, your subconscious may be programmed to watch for movement in your peripheral vision. Even if you are not consciously thinking about or looking for mice, your subconscious will still be on the lookout for this 'threat'.

If the threat is always present and cannot be avoided (if, for example, you have to work with mice), you may feel the threat subconsciously even if you aren't consciously focused on it. You will then be in a heightened state of alertness without realising it.

Skilled filmmakers use these techniques to keep audiences on edge without clearly identifying the source of the angst. You may have experienced this unexplained uneasy feeling from time to time.

Cognitive behaviour therapy is a common tool used by psychologists to deal with worry and fears. The patient talks about the problem to examine its meaning and threat rationally. My hope is that PECs reading this book will already have done this by understanding the problem. If you realise that your concern about your illness reinforces the ANS dysfunction, then you don't have to be worried about some other mysterious unexplained cause of your symptoms or other threat. When you realise that the worry is the threat, you will be able to stop it more easily. You can choose to stop it, not only because there is nothing to worry about, but because you cannot afford to do so any longer.

You can use many techniques to achieve this. **The key thing is to interrupt the focus on symptoms and the anticipation of potential symptoms. Instead, shift your focus to something else, like a good novel, jobs around the house, or dreams of a vacation you can enjoy once you are well.**

You may also get help from an experienced psychologist, counsellor, hypnotherapist, NLP and TimeLine Therapist, or other practitioner.

The chicken-or-egg conundrum:

What comes first, full restoration of health (ending the symptoms that help cause the ANS dysfunction) or the total correction of the ANS dysfunction (that causes the symptoms)?

As we've said, if you continue to look for and treat symptoms, you will likely perpetuate the ANS dysfunction. But if you don't treat severe secondary dysfunctions, then ignoring them may be difficult and the physical dysfunctions themselves may trigger the ANS.

PECs who recovered by focussing solely on the mental side of things often recommend shifting attention away from symptoms and to eliminate conscious and subconscious concern about them. But this alone won't work for many people because mental and emotional stress due to the symptoms are only one of their triggers. That's why I prefer a holistic, multilateral approach that includes both brain training and physical strategies.

But doing both may be too much of a balancing act for some. The reason is that whilst you are trying other treatments and monitoring symptoms to see if they're effective, you are reinforcing the ANS dysfunction. This sabotages your efforts.

So, if symptoms are severe, it may be better for some people to focus first on physical treatments and lifestyle changes. Once severe imbalances and dysfunctions have been addressed, I recommend that you continue with your diet, lifestyle, and basic supplement regimes but focus on ANS normalisation through brain training.

3. Mental and emotional stress from the environment (conscious and subconscious)

As I've said, most people know that mental stress triggers their symptoms and makes them worse, so we know it is a key issue. However, some mental or emotional stressors may not be clearly identified or easy to deal with. Here are some stresses to consider:

- Excessive mental or physical workload
- Inability to meet basic needs for shelter, clothing, and food
- Insecurity about your ability to continue to meet these needs

- Inability to meet needs of love, intimacy, or belonging

Here are some more specific examples:

- Marital problems
- Conflict or bullying
- Abuse of any kind or violence
- Financial pressures or failure
- Loss of a loved one
- The pressures of caring for sick people

Another prevalent source of stress for PECs is of course dealing with CFS itself. We have already discussed worry about illness and symptoms, but the impact of having CFS is often severe. It places pressure on major aspects of life such as relationships, finances, and the ability to meet basic needs. (That is why I wrote *Discover Hope*, a short book designed to help people cope with CFS and find a more productive and positive attitude for their recovery journey.)

You cannot wave a magic wand and make these stressors disappear. However, if you realise they are physically harming you—keeping you sick—you may get enough mental leverage to make some tough decisions, or at least to get help to overcome some of these problems. **When we cannot remove problems, we can still change how we deal with them and what meaning we give to them.**

Some sources of subconscious emotional stress can be subtle and difficult to identify. Speaking with a trained counsellor or psychologist may be helpful, as they may help you pinpoint the problem and identify unaddressed feelings and issues. Be careful not to focus too much on the past. In my opinion, spending your life discussing your history may not serve you. Express unexpressed emotions, deal with unidentified problems, and then move on with your life. The right trained counsellor or psychologist can be very helpful with this.

A diary can also be valuable in identifying sources of stress. If you notice that you seem to get sick whenever you have a meeting with your boss or get a phone call from your sister, then you may have to address this. In some circumstances, you may have to make drastic changes, but in others, you may just have to reframe the issue. You should walk through this process with the help of an objective person who has your best interests at heart. The problem may lie less with the other person's behaviour than with your interpretation of it or your way of dealing with it.

Before you quit your job or disown a family member, learn to make changes. It's usually more productive and helpful, in the short and long term, to be more assertive, calmly express your feelings, and ask others to stop certain behaviours. Sometimes we just need a little space for a short time, so ask for that respectfully.

As your ANS dysfunction normalises and your physical and mental resources increase, you will find that you no longer need to be on autopilot. You will regain your judgement and your ability to choose your responses wisely. Few things will help you achieve this more than daily mindfulness meditation practice.

4. Mental and emotional stress experienced in the past (conscious and subconscious)

We are all likely to have some emotional and mental stress in our past. Whilst we may not have fully dealt with these, I don't think they will necessarily cause CFS or stop you from recovering. However, if the mental or emotional stress was traumatic and has not been dealt with, it may be sufficient to perpetuate CFS.

Do look at any significant life event that occurred immediately prior to your illness. Whilst you may feel that you have already dealt with it, if tears well up when you speak about it in detail with someone, you may have a bit more work to do.

If you suspect you are in this category, speak with a qualified counsellor or psychologist to identify this event. You might also consider alternative therapies such as Neuro-Linguistic Programming (NLP) or TimeLine Therapy to complement your other counselling.

Another trigger of
the ANS dysfunction

Clearly, the four primary triggers of the ANS dysfunction must be addressed. But there is another trigger; the ANS dysfunction itself.

As we've seen, arousal is a self-perpetuating condition. Arousal and hypervigilance are significant causes of stress in their own right. They may skew your approach to other life challenges and your stress response to them.

Becoming aware of inappropriate stress reactions

Have you ever been in a really heated argument—and then someone else asked a simple question and you snapped at them? In the heat of the moment, when our arousal is high, our emotions are so strong that even a simple problem like "I can't find the stapler" or "Mummy, can I do my painting now?" can be too much. We snap.

Let's review the definition of stress: a response to a gap, real or perceived, between a demand and the ability to meet that demand.

Some stress can boost your performance. However, excessive stress is likely to diminish your performance significantly. Your diminished performance can then widen the gap between demands and your ability to meet them. This, by definition, is further stress, and it can cause a downward spiral.

This means that the things that your unstressed self could have handled in a calm and intelligent manner are suddenly too much for you. And the consequences of not dealing with them effectively are usually further problems—further sources of stress.

When stress and your arousal levels have been high for an extended period of time, you may not even be aware of them anymore. You may do everything with an underlying simmering of emotions that explode to the surface quickly and easily.

Once you become aware of this problem, you may realise that you are holding your breath or tensing your muscles whilst performing even simple tasks, let alone any that involve physical exertion. And performing physical actions whilst holding your breath further interferes with your performance. It is clearly stressful.

When you realise that you are bracing your body, holding your breath, hunching your shoulders, or tensing your neck—feeling stressed or getting overexcited—**interrupt the pattern.** Take a breath, relax, and try to continue more effectively. This takes a little practice, especially at first.

Reducing your baseline arousal levels

The key to moving forward is to reduce your arousal. There are many ways of doing this indirectly like listening to music, going for a leisurely walk in the country, relaxing at the beach, or reading a good book with no rush or agenda.

However, in my opinion, one of the best ways to reduce your arousal is meditation. Meditation does not have to be a religious practice, although most religions including Christianity, Islam, Buddhism, and Hinduism practice prayer that is akin to meditation. The idea of meditation is to learn to still your mind and practice holding it still. Over time, it becomes easier and your baseline arousal drops.

It may not stop your SNS from triggering the fight-or-flight response, but it will help you become more aware of when it happens. Then you can down-regulate this response by triggering your PNS.

There are many different forms of meditation and many different programs available. Try several and go with what works for you and what you enjoy. Make sure you persist even though it may initially be a little difficult.

In my experience, what works best for PECs is mindfulness meditation skewed towards letting go or defocusing. Rigid focussing meditation may sometimes have negative effects on sensitive PECs in my view.

Avoid overstimulation

During your recovery, stay away from television as much as possible, especially movies that are stimulating, fast-moving, or loud, or that depict strong negative themes like sadness, anger, or violence. Also avoid news and current affair programs, which are mostly negative.

Music can be very relaxing, but it can also be stimulating, so choose your music carefully. Heavy metal or hip hop music may not be your best choice early on. Something slow and soothing (even boring) is more suitable.

Aim to strike a balance. If going to a football game gives you lot of enjoyment and helps you focus on something positive, that's fantastic. But don't overdo it.

Pain desensitisation & dealing with specific triggers

Pain is both a symptom and a trigger. It could arguably have been included in either of the first trigger categories:

1. Physical stress due to bodily dysfunctions (subconscious) OR
2. Mental and emotional stress about CFS and its symptoms (conscious and subconscious)

Given that the brain has learned to feel pain at inappropriate excessive levels, it goes to follow that the brain can also unlearn this. Indeed research in the latter half of the twentieth century has proven that the brain is plastic (able to change). This has led to amazing medical breakthroughs, such as cochlear implants that have allowed people to hear again, or even to hear for the first time.

But how can the brain learn this? How can we achieve pain **desensitisation**?

The key is **normalising ANS function and brain arousal**. This allows the brain to restore our hormone and neurotransmitter levels. It also reduces any secondary causes of pain, such as inflammation.

Surprisingly, psychological factors are involved in pain perception. We all understand some of these factors intuitively, like when we distract our children the moment before ripping off a bandage. These various factors create the opportunity for brain retraining to reduce pain.

A skilled pain psychologist can help you explore these factors as part of your overall recovery process. If you cannot find somebody who specializes in pain normalisation or desensitisation, then look for a pain management class. Whilst its aim may sound more modest, the underlying processes are often the same.

Moreover, the techniques that you learn to retrain your nervous systems response to other symptoms also apply to pain. Just as you change how you pay attention, anticipate and feel about your other symptoms, making such changes to pain will be helpful not just with ANS normalisation, but also pain desensitisation.

You may also notice that certain other things trigger your CFS symptoms. These may be arguments, crowded environments, the smell of chemicals, exposure to electromagnetic radiation or sun, noise, or vibrations.

Whilst you should avoid stressful situations where possible, triggers actually offer a great opportunity to normalise your ANS. You can recondition your nervous system by switching on your PNS and relaxing during the exposure. I don't suggest that you specifically seek out these triggers, but when you come across them, clear your mind of panic or worry, acknowledge the sensation, and practice relaxing. This may take some time to achieve, and coaching by an experienced professional may be helpful.

Final thoughts on ANS normalisation

Making these changes can take a little time, although for some people they can be surprisingly quick. You may be surprised to see that you have been living in a continually stressed state. In fact, the trauma of having CFS may catch up with you at this point. Talking about it with a counsellor can be a very good idea, especially if you have been sick for a longer period of time.

Do consider seeking help from a meditation teacher, counsellor, psychologist, hypnotherapist, or NLP or TimeLine Therapy Practitioner.

Focus your therapy on overcoming any fears of specific triggers as well as general fears about having CFS.

CHAPTER SUMMARY

- The ANS dysfunction is an inappropriate and ongoing stress response to a variety of triggers.
- The four main causes of the ANS dysfunction are:
  - Stress due to bodily dysfunctions (subconscious)
  - Stress and concern about the illness and symptoms of CFS (conscious and subconscious)
  - Mental and emotional stress experienced in your current environment (conscious and subconscious)
  - Mental and emotional stress experienced in your past (conscious and subconscious)
- Another cause is the ANS dysfunction itself. To overcome this you need to do the following:
  - Become aware of inappropriate stress reactions and interrupt these patterns.
  - Reduce your baseline level of arousal.
- If pain is an issue, seek the help of a pain psychologist for pain management or desensitisation training.
- The following things may be helpful in reducing your arousal levels:
  - Meditating daily
  - Going for leisurely walks in nature
  - Listening to music
  - Reading a relaxing book
  - Avoiding stimulating things like exciting movies or the news

CHAPTER 17

A Diet to Thrive On

"The human body heals itself and nutrition provides the resources to accomplish the task."

- Roger Williams, Ph.D.

Why bother with diet?

Despite the old adage "You are what you eat," I never considered the role of food during all my years of illness. After all, other people had much worse diets than I did and they weren't sick.

CFS isn't caused by poor diet alone. So why is diet so important?

I am reminded of another statement I have heard people say, "You replace every cell in your body every seven years."

Whilst this is not strictly true, every cell in your body relies on the nutrients that you take in: oils to build cell membranes, minerals for chemical reactions to produce energy, proteins and cholesterol to build hormones and neurotransmitters. Your cells need countless other substances as well, many of which are not fully understood. We know, for example, that spinach has carbohydrates and minerals that the body needs, but what about the hundreds of phytonutrients that help prevent cell damage and cancer cell replication and that decrease cholesterol levels?

You are made up of trillions of cells. Each cell relies on what you eat to perform the almost unimaginably complex functions that make up the human body. Each cell may also be affected negatively by what you drink, eat, or ingest by breathing or skin absorption.

Food matters, a lot. But what is the right diet for PECs—or for anyone, for that matter?

Few choices in our world today are as confusing as what foods to eat or avoid. Everybody says something different. No other animal seems to have this problem.

Perhaps the simple answer is too much choice. As little as 20,000 years ago, humans didn't have this problem. They ate whatever they found that was edible. But these days many of our choices are so far from natural that many people don't know the difference between natural and processed foods.

Food should be simple, but these days there are many problems with it. Making the right choices becomes complicated, especially when you have a multi-systemic illness such as CFS.

Let me start by impressing upon you that **your choice of food is critical.** For many years I made the mistake of underestimating the power of food, both for healing and for causing disease. If an engine starts to lose power, blow smoke, or make noise, the first things you will check are the fuel and oil. You will make sure they are of the right type and quality. But many of us don't give food the respect it deserves. I believe the reason is that the impact of the wrong food is usually not immediate. We can appear healthy for years eating a diet that doesn't meet our needs. It's only when our reserves are drained or our systems are pushed over a stress threshold that something 'suddenly' goes wrong.

Food can be your biggest poison or your best medicine. Ignore this most important aspect of your treatment at your peril. Many people overcome or slow down even 'terminal' illnesses simply by changing their diet. These healings are usually called unexplained or spontaneous remissions.

It is important to realise that PECs are **severely** dysfunctional and that each case is different. PECs need to carefully consider their diets and, to some extent, tailor it to their specific needs. They may have to readjust it from time to time to overcome particular obstacles or to meet different objectives. Diets may include the following:

- Anti-gut-allergy/-inflammation diet, eliminating dairy and wheat products.
- Anti-hypoglycaemia diet, low in sugar products such as soft drinks, milk, confectionaries, processed foods, flour products, and rice; may also limit high sugar fruits such as melons, grapes, and dried fruits.
- Anti-candida diet, similar to an anti-hypoglycaemia diet but also eliminating yeast, alcohol, and most fermented products, as well as dairy and wheat.
- Detoxification diet, similar to the above, but may include extra proteins and important supplements.
- Muscle and nervous system rehabilitation diet, targeting specific amino acids and B vitamins.
- Trace mineral balancing diet, including foods that contain particular trace minerals.

There are many possible choices. Trying to discuss all of them here would make for an extremely long book and would likely confuse or overwhelm you.

The solution is to find a coach, such as a holistic doctor or a naturopath, to **fine tune your diet**. For example, if you are suffering severe adrenal insufficiency and your sodium–potassium balance is off, you can increase your salt intake and temporarily decrease your intake of potassium-rich foods.

And whilst you may need a low-carbohydrate or low-protein diet early on, as your activity picks up and your muscles rehabilitate, you will need to make adjustments. It makes sense to start with a good base diet and then adjust it by listening to your body and getting advice as you need it.

Remember to make adjustments gradually. They should not be extreme. Cutting out all carbohydrates or all protein or all fat is not only difficult and unhelpful, it may be dangerous.

In this chapter, I describe a good base diet—not the 'best' diet or the 'perfect' diet. The best diet for a very healthy person may not be the best diet for a sick one. Each person has different needs.

Eating a better diet is a practical thing that you can do now to address some of your main problems and create a good base for recovery.

A note for vegetarians or vegans

If you are a vegetarian or vegan for religious, ethical, or health reasons, I completely understand. Even if we ignore the ethical considerations in how animals are raised and slaughtered, the quality of much meat is questionable. Besides making the body acidic, too much meat may also increase its toxic burden.

My biggest concern for vegans and vegetarians is not so much the lack of protein and vitamin B12 (although this is an issue for PECs), but what you eat *instead* of animal products. A diet composed chiefly of processed foods, unfermented soy products, and grain products such as bread and pasta is not supportive of recovery!

All people—especially PECs—need a healthy and supportive diet that provides the required nutrients for the body without creating toxic exposure, excess acid, or inflammation in the body.

However, cutting out any food group means that your diet needs to be that much better. If you also reduce carbohydrate sources such as grains, bread, pasta, white potatoes, and rice, you may be left with serious nutritional deficiencies and insufficient calories.

Vegetarians and vegans must seek advice to tailor a diet to their specific needs. Consider the guidelines in this book under the advice of a nutritionist or qualified doctor or naturopath. You might also need to consider eating a greater variety of foods for a period of time.

What are you trying to achieve with your diet?

Let's first list some of the challenges of CFS on which diet will have the most impact.

- Hypoglycaemia and insulin resistance
- Toxic accumulation and detoxification problems
- Mineral imbalances
- Gut problems, including poor gut function, leaky gut, candida, poor gut flora, or parasites
- Poor cellular function
- Excessive inflammation
- Neurotransmitter imbalances

Another way of looking at the foods you eat is how acidic or alkaline they make your body. Numerous books have been written about this, so I'll just say that an alkaline environment is desirable and an acidic one is not. That does not mean that you should *only* eat foods that are alkalising; extreme diets do not make sense and can be harmful.

Diet alone will not fix mineral imbalances, but it can certainly make them better or worse. For example, PECs whose sodium–potassium balance is off need to pay particular attention to foods that are very rich in sodium or potassium.

As your challenges are addressed, your naturopath or holistic doctor may change your diet and add certain supplements for a period of time. This chapter includes guidelines for normalising blood sugar and cortisol response, for rebuilding the body's cellular and glandular health, and for reducing inflammation.

Before I discuss when, how, and what to eat, let me ask my favourite question: *Why?*

I believe that CFS is caused by a disruption in the regulation of the ANS. This leads to periods of excessive and then insufficient cortisol which causes many bodily dysfunctions. These include mitochondrial dysfunction, poor blood sugar regulation, immune dysfunction, gut dysfunction, fatigue, and other hormone and neurotransmitter imbalances.

Another problem is direct nervous system stimulation (or lack of it) for systems of the body such as the cardiovascular and digestive systems.

As we've discussed, one of the four primary triggers of the ANS dysfunction is physical stress due to bodily dysfunctions. This subconscious stress can be due to things such as poor blood sugar regulation, toxic stress, hormonal malfunctioning, and so on.

Diet can directly impact this triggering, by creating toxic stress, affecting hydration levels, and contributing to hormonal and neurotransmitter imbalances.

However, hypoglycaemic episodes may have the biggest impact on the ANS dysfunction. So **maintaining a healthy blood sugar level is critical.** Down-regulating the ANS dysfunction by other means is also critical, but physical activity and food impact blood sugar levels directly. That is why you must focus on diet as part of your recovery.

The five pillars of the CFS recovery diet

1. Avoid food and drinks that lead to blood glucose surges

Few things are more important to your wellbeing than stopping the rollercoaster ride of plunging blood sugar levels and damaging insulin surges. Let's consider in more detail how foods impact our body.

Three broad categories of nutrients provide energy: protein, fat, and carbohydrates. Carbohydrates impact our blood sugar most directly, so we should first focus on them. Carbohydrates are changed into glucose (blood sugar). The speed at which this happens depends on how much change has to occur to turn them into glucose molecules.

Simple carbohydrates turn into sugars the fastest. These include the sugar in confectioneries, cakes, and other sweet desserts. They also include fruit. Reaching for a bunch of grapes instead of a candy bar won't improve your sugar rollercoaster a whole lot. Fruit is great in terms of vitamins, minerals, and other nutrients. However, **if you must eat sweet fruits that rapidly convert to glucose, you should eat them in small portions, as part of a meal, along with other fats and proteins to reduce the impact of the sugar.** Sweet fruits include bananas, dates, grapes, melons, mangoes, nectarines, oranges, papayas, pineapples, plums, pomegranates, tangerines, and all dried fruit. Other fruit should be eaten in moderation during your recovery. The exceptions are low-sugar fruits such as avocado, cucumbers, tomatoes, eggplant, zucchini, and capsicum, which you can eat in substantial amounts.

Next on the list are starchy carbohydrates. These are foods like grains, potatoes, sweet potato, carrots, peas, pumpkin and corn. Grains can be unrefined or refined. Refined grains are reduced to nothing but the starchy part. Examples of refined grains are white flour and white rice. It is best to avoid them as well as any products made from them (such as pasta, bread and other baked goods). Similarly, you should avoid white potatoes, although *moderate* servings of sweet potatoes, pumpkin, corn, peas, and cooked carrots are fine. Raw carrots are also fine to eat and have less of an impact than cooked carrots.

Other sources of carbohydrates **are low-carb or non-starchy vegetables.** These are greens such as lettuce, spinach, chard, collards, kale, herbs, bok choy, bamboo shoots, celery, cabbage, brussels sprouts, and asparagus, as well as edible flowers such as cauliflower and broccoli. **You should eat these whenever possible, in plentiful amounts.**

You can probably guess that drinking cola and other soft drinks that have high sugar contents is a bad idea. But you should also realise that drinking fruit juice or milk will send your blood sugar soaring. Fruit juice is full of a sugar called fructose. Whilst fructose has a less direct impact on blood glucose, it increases insulin resistance and bad cholesterol, places an extra burden on your liver. Fruit juice often has as much or more sugar than soft drinks such as cola. Milk sugar (lactose) is not much better. Adding sugar, honey, or milk to hot drinks such as coffee and tea will also spike your blood sugar.

The following are five things you must avoid during recovery:
- White bread and any pasta
- White potatoes and white rice
- Sweets
- Sugary drinks, including juice
- Alcohol (discussed in the next section)

---

2. Avoid stimulants and toxins

PECs need to get their detox mechanisms working again. It's obvious, then, that ingesting extra toxins is a bad idea, but we may not always be aware of which things are toxins or stimulants.

Stimulants

The most common stimulants are coffee and tea, which you should eliminate from your diet. (You may, however, drink non-stimulating herbal teas.) You should also avoid hot chocolate, which contains sugar as well as caffeine.

Energy drinks are absolute poison to PECs, as they are high in sugar and often in caffeine and other stimulants.

Because caffeine is a drug, it is important that you do not withdraw from it too quickly, especially if your cortisol regulation is highly dysfunctional. Withdrawal symptoms only last a few days for most people, but PECs who rely heavily on caffeine may be strongly affected. I suggest a gradual withdrawal, over a week or two.

Social Poisons

Alcohol is a special poison, given that PECs have a low tolerance for it. Whilst it may cause an initial increase in blood sugar, depending on the type of drink, it is followed by a plunge in blood sugar that leads to the cortisol response that we are trying to minimise. **Alcohol is absolutely taboo for PECs until they have recovered.**

Smoking is one of the most serious toxic exposures we can have. Cigarette smoke doesn't just include tar, nicotine, and dozens of cancer-causing chemicals; it also includes hundreds of toxins. These enter your bloodstream, burden every cell in your body, and put extra pressure on your liver. Reduce or eliminate your exposure where possible.

I hope it goes without saying that other recreational drugs are also taboo. First, they add to your toxic burden. Second, interference with an already malfunctioning nervous system and out-of-balance hormonal and neurotransmitter levels can have drastic and undesired effects.

Pesticide Poisons

Another source of toxins is meat, fish, fruit, and vegetables. Many factory farm animals are exposed to significant amounts of toxins. Fruits and vegetables are sprayed with a large range of poisons. These all add to the toxic burden.

Going totally organic may not be within your means. However, a few guidelines can help you reduce the toxic burden of your food if you can't buy organics.

Meat
- Buy lean, wild meats where possible.
- Buy meat from grass fed animals.
- Avoid eating the fat in meat, especially in non-organic meat.

Seafood
- Avoid fish high in the food chain, such as king mackerel, shark, tuna, grouper, and swordfish.
- Avoid long-lived fish, such as orange roughy.
- Avoid buying fish imported from countries with polluted waters.

Fruits and vegetables
- Buy organic whenever possible.
- If your budget does not allow for organic produce, consider the research compiled by the US Environmental Working Group

(EWG) from approximately 51,000 tests of 53 popular fruits and vegetables. EWG suggests that eating five servings of fruit and vegetables from the cleanest fifteen fruits and vegetables, rather than the most contaminated twelve ('the dirty dozen'), will reduce your pesticide exposure by 92%.

- The amount of pesticide in non-organic vegetables differs, depending on the country they are grown in. Consider the sources of the food you buy. Developing countries in Asia and South America may have different safety standards.

Table 2 below puts fruits and vegetables into three categories: those that should always come from organic sources; those that may be less harmful if not organic; and finally, those that may have only small amounts of pesticide residue.

	Eat in quantity during recovery	Eat sparingly during recovery	Eat in small amounts after recovery
ALWAYS BUY ORGANIC	Celery Spinach Capsicum (sweet bell peppers) Lettuce Kale Cucumbers	Apples Strawberries Peaches Nectarines Blueberries Cherries Raspberries	Beets Grapes Parsnips Swede
BUY ORGANIC WHERE POSSIBLE	Carrots (raw) Summer squash/ zucchini Green beans Broccoli Green onions Cauliflower Tomatoes	Sweet potatoes Pears Plums Oranges Cranberries Honeydew Melon Grapefruit Papaya	Carrots (cooked) Bananas Cantaloupe Winter squash/ pumpkins Mushrooms
BUY ORGANIC WHERE NOT TOO COSTLY	Asparagus Avocados Cabbage Onions Sweet peas	Kiwis Eggplants	Watermelon Pineapple Mango Sweet corn

Table 2 : Organic Vegetable/Fruit Guide

I have not included white potatoes in this chart, as I believe they are one vegetable that everyone should avoid. They have a very high glycaemic index and cause a strong insulin response. If you must eat potatoes, buy organic ones, as non-organic white potatoes are one of the most pesticide-ridden vegetables on the market.

Fat and Oil Poisons

Fat and oils have been vilified, sometimes unjustly, in my opinion. The key is which fats and oils you choose and how you use them. For example, a good oil, like olive oil, when heated to a high temperature, can become a bad oil.

Let me say, without going into the full discussion on fats and oils, that different ones can offer significant health benefits or hazards. They are often categorised as saturated or unsaturated fats. Saturated fats come primarily from animals; most consider them to be 'bad'. Unsaturated fats come from plants; most people consider them to be 'good'. **This is a gross oversimplification and not correct.**

Whilst eating too much saturated fat can have negative impacts, I believe that one of the biggest concerns is processed foods and a third fat group that they contain called trans fats. Trans fats are unsaturated fats that have been chemically altered to become saturated fats through a process called hydrogenation. This process has been around for a little over a hundred years. Cookies, chips, donuts, crackers, candy, salad dressings, and even breakfast cereals can all contain trans fats. Trans fats impact health negatively and have been implicated in major diseases. **Trans fats are not natural** (only small amounts exist in natural foods) **and you should avoid them.**

Whilst unsaturated oils sound good, many can easily go rancid. They are oxidised in your body, causing inflammation and disturbing the endocrine system. I believe that **canola, cottonseed, corn, safflower, sunflower, and soybean oils are all to be avoided. Vegetable shortening and margarine should also be avoided.**

So what should you eat? First, don't eat oil, eat food. Food should not be deep fried. If you have to fry something, use butter or coconut oil. These should not be eaten in large amounts because they are saturated fats, but that makes them stable at high temperatures. They are therefore a better option than other oils for high-heat cooking.

If you have to use a spread on bread, use butter in small amounts. Better still, use nut butters, hummus, or avocado. (Don't use peanut butter; peanuts are not actually nuts.) Remember, we don't want to eat too much bread anyway.

If you want to add oil to salads or other foods, olive oil is best. Just make sure that you don't use it for cooking. Buy cold-pressed, virgin olive oil, and store it in a cool place out of direct light.

We store a lot of toxins in our body fat. So do animals. Always eat low-fat meat, and trim off fat whenever possible.

3. Focus on eating vegetables

Eat vegetables, vegetables, and more vegetables. Find ones you like, and invent ways to enjoy the ones you don't. **Low-sugar vegetables and fruits should be the focus for your recovery.**

In stir fries and salads, as sides, as snacks—whenever you can, eat low-sugar vegetables and fruits. No, man cannot live on vegetables alone, so add fat and proteins such as nuts, eggs, and small amounts of good-quality meat and fish.

Nuts and seeds are a great snack. They are packed with protein, fatty acids, vitamins, minerals, enzymes, and antioxidants. Good choices include almonds, Brazil nuts, hazelnuts, macadamias, pecans, pine nuts, pumpkin seeds, sunflower seeds, and walnuts. Avoid peanuts, which are highly allergenic. Pistachios and cashews may have mould and may not be the best choice for PECs. The most important thing is that the nuts are raw and fresh. They should ideally be stored in a sealed container, in a refrigerator or freezer to keep them from going rancid.

4. Prepare your food wisely

To avoid pesticides, I urge you to wash fruits and vegetables thoroughly with a vegetable wash that breaks up wax, soil, and waterproof agricultural chemicals. Ask for this at your local health food store or check the Internet. Whilst some may disagree, I think it also makes sense to peel conventionally-grown fruits and vegetables. It is worth losing some of the nutrients in order to reduce your exposure to harmful chemicals.

Wash the food first, then peel and rinse. However, you should realise that **washing and peeling conventionally-grown fruits and vegetables will not entirely remove pesticides**.

Prepare food in batches. If you have to wash and peel and cut just to have a quick snack, you are more likely to grab something convenient and processed that's full of carbohydrates and trans fats.

Where possible, eat vegetables raw. If you have to cook them, steam or boil them lightly. Eating vegetables raw ensures that they are not damaged by heat and that the nutrients are not lost in the cooking water.

One of the best sources of water for our bodies is from fresh, raw, organic vegetables and low-sugar fruits that contain valuable minerals, vitamins and enzymes.

I believe you should eat both cooked and raw food. Some authors claim that when you cook food, you make around 50% of the protein unavailable and destroy 60-70% of the vitamins, virtually all the vitamin B12 and 100% of the phytonutrients. (If you are eating meat to get vitamin B12, this could be a problem.) Others say that cooking food makes some nutrients more bio-available.

Obviously, most fish and meat needs to be cooked, as do many root vegetables. However, the impact of cooking on enzymes and phytonutrients is not yet well understood.

One of the healthiest methods of cooking for fish, meat and eggs is poaching. If you have to fry or bake, use small amounts of coconut oil or butter.

I recommend that you avoid microwaves. Microwaved vegetables may look better than vegetables cooked in a pot, because boiling them leaches out colour as well as nutrients. However, concerns have been raised over the safety of microwaved food (although this is still a controversial issue). Using the wrong dishware can add toxic substances to the food, and many nutrients lose their value. Minerals appear unaffected, but many antioxidants, proteins, and vitamins lose their bioavailability.

The Germans invented microwave ovens for their troops during World War II; the Russians investigated the technology after the war. Both groups found real concerns, chiefly the production of carcinogenic substances when food is irradiated by microwave radiation. The Russians banned the use of microwave ovens in 1976 due to health concerns, although the ban was later lifted.

5. When, how, and what to eat

One of the main objectives of the diet is to reduce hypoglycaemic episodes that trigger the HPA axis.

At first, the timing of your eating may have the biggest impact on blood sugar regulation. As with anything to do with health, there are many conflicting opinions. Should you graze all day long or eat one large meal a day? Should you have periods of fasting and feasting or take in a steady and regular stream of calories?

The answer depends on a few things. But PECs who have hypoglycaemic episodes should eat regularly, in small amounts. The ideal is regular, small, balanced meals and snacks that are low in simple carbohydrates and that have some fat and protein.

Your first and last meals of the day may be the most important, given the role of cortisol in blood sugar regulation. Since you don't eat during sleep, in the morning your glycogen reserves are depleted. To counter this, your cortisol levels should rise sharply.

However, if your cortisol levels are low because of adrenal insufficiency, your blood sugar will remain low. Your body will try to produce cortisol to avert a crisis, but you will feel terribly low in energy. You are also stressing your body and triggering your HPA axis. This will further sensitise your overactive ANS.

I believe it's essential to eat a balanced breakfast soon after waking (and no later than 9:00 am), even if you don't feel like it. It is essential that it contain protein, some complex carbohydrates, and some fat. If your liver is congested, eating eggs—or anything—early in the day may be a real struggle. However, do persist. If you can't eat eggs, try an easy-to-digest, vegetable- or nut-based alternative.

Make sure that you avoid high-sugar breakfasts like cereal with milk which are likely to be poorly tolerated by your digestive system. These are likely to spike your blood sugar and insulin, and they will not help normalise your gut function or bowel habits. Dropping the cereal-and-milk breakfast may be one of the best changes you can make. Consider making it permanent, even after you have recovered from CFS.

Both lunch and dinner should be eaten early, around 11:30 am and 5:30pm respectively, before your blood sugar drops too much. Again, these meals should include a balance of carbohydrates, fats, and protein.

Snacking between meals, especially in the afternoon, is important to keep your blood sugar levels steady and avoid an energy lull that might make you reach for a sugary snack or cup of coffee. Even a bad snack may be better than no snack at all, but try to have a quality snack and avoid stimulants like coffee. Stimulants may make you feel better at first, but they trigger your HPA axis, which is what we are trying to avoid. Instead, have a low-glycaemic, balanced snack that keeps you fuelled until your next meal.

Just before you start your bedtime routine, have a small, low-carbohydrate snack with protein. This will help you get through the night without triggering your HPA axis and waking you up. It will also help rebuild important hormones and neurotransmitters.

Most importantly, enjoy your food. This is not about deprivation, so make the effort to make your meals tasty. Discover new foods and food combinations, and give yourself the time to eat it in a slow and relaxed manner. The benefits of eating slowly, chewing well, and being in a relaxed state are well known. They form an important part of your eating plan.

From theory to practice: some meal examples

Breakfast

My favourite choices include one slice of dark, wholemeal rye bread with seeds, spread thickly with avocado, topped with a little tuna or salmon and plenty of quality sea salt. You might also have a poached or boiled egg with a piece of rye toast and a fresh, salted tomato. If you have more time, you can make a salad of tomatoes, cucumbers, a little apple, and avocado, sprinkled with raw almonds and macadamias; dress it with sea salt, virgin olive oil, and a dash of apple cider vinegar or lemon juice. (Yum!)

Use your imagination. Think fresh and balanced. Once you are used to making these breakfasts, you will find that the extra five to ten minutes of preparation are well worth it, both in how much you enjoy the food and in how you feel afterwards.

You may also be surprised at the many foods which initially sound strange and unappetising that turn out to be delicious and nutritious. One example is a small serving of brown rice (ideally cooked the day before) heated in a saucepan with half a chopped apple, some almonds and seeds, and a small amount of nut butter and nut mylk. Warm this mixture through, but don't boil it. Top it off with fresh berries. It's really delicious.

Lunch and dinner

Lightly-steamed or raw vegetables are great. For a cooked meal, serve grilled fish or poached chicken with a large serving of lightly-cooked or raw brightly-coloured vegetables. If you need carbohydrates, try a small palm-sized serving of brown or wild rice or a small amount of sweet potato. If you must have bread, have a small slice of wholemeal rye or another low- or non-wheat bread. Stay away from pasta or potatoes. Feel free to add a little fat to your meal, ideally uncooked olive oil, avocado, or an occasional drizzle of butter.

Also try options such as lentil curry or bean chilli, but go easy on these whilst your digestive system is still irritable. Eat them with a serving of greens and sometimes with a little brown rice.

Soups are an excellent option. Make sure you add a little protein so that afterwards you are not hungry and looking for unhealthy snacks.

Wraps made from wholemeal rye let you eat plenty of vegetables without too many high-glycaemic carbohydrates. For moisture and flavour, add a little yogurt or a dash of chilli sauce (not too much as this is very sugary). You can also add cottage cheese, eggs, or quality fish or meat for protein, to help you feel satisfied and full.

Between-meal snacks

Fresh raw nuts are an excellent choice to nibble on throughout the day. Ideally, you should buy or make a mix of nuts and seeds, to give you a good mix of nutrients. Avoid mixes with dried fruit. If you have a small piece of fresh fruit (say, half an apple or pear), make sure that you eat some nuts first.

Another option is wholemeal rye crackers with avocado or raw carrot and celery, with hummus or nut butters.

Remember to drink plenty of water.

Bedtime snacks

Bedtime snacks should be small, with good fat and protein and only a small amount of complex carbohydrates. Snacks with simple carbs or too many carbs can be counterproductive and keep you awake.

Some examples are raw carrot or other vegetable sticks with cottage cheese; a wholemeal rye cracker with a little nut butter or hummus (not too much); or a boiled egg with gherkins.

Treats

The habit of eating a rich desert after a meal is a recent phenomenon. It is not normal, healthy or natural. If you currently eat like this, I recommend that you try to change your eating habits.

However, you will probably want to treat yourself now and then. Even daily treats are okay if eaten in moderation. **I recommend that**

you maximise the flavour and satisfaction to minimise the sugar content.

Dark chocolate is an excellent choice. Once you are used to the taste, you will never want to go back to milk chocolate. You should only have a small piece, not a whole bar. You need only a small amount to get the satisfaction you are seeking, and eating slowly is more satisfying. In fact, you will probably find that normal chocolate is a letdown in comparison. Normal chocolate is usually very high in sugar, and you will often eat more than you should, so I recommend that you avoid this and other confectionaries.

Make sure you avoid high-carbohydrate baked goods. In my experience, foods that have a strong taste, with some fat but few carbohydrates, are the best. They can be enjoyed in small quantities and still be satisfying.

Treats based on coconut and nuts may be good options. If you don't make them yourself, check the quality. Baked goods can be made using nut flours instead of wheat flour. They may be filled with fruit and nuts or even some quark or mascarpone cheese. You might also try a small amount of fruit with whipped cream, or a small piece of custard tart for an occasional treat.

But it's best to learn to live without daily sugar rushes.

Once you are well: the ultimate diet

When you are almost fully recovered, you might want to consider a champion diet that lays the foundations for lasting health. Because this diet is not initially appropriate for PECs, I won't go into detail, but let me give you some guidelines for future research.

Grains and grain products may have had one of the biggest negative impacts on human health. This is a recent phenomenon, as humans did not regularly consume grains for hundreds of thousands of years. Consuming them robs you of minerals in several ways, causes inflammation due to high omega-6 fatty acid content, and breaks down the microvilli in your small intestine (which can cause leaky gut syndrome). They also contain allergenic proteins called lectins that play havoc with your immune system.

However, a diet totally without grains takes careful planning and a big change in eating habits, and in my opinion, it is not ideal for PECs. If your body is not conditioned to metabolise fatty acids and proteins well enough, such a low-carbohydrate diet could cause hypoglycaemia—the very thing you are trying to avoid. However, whilst you are recovering, a gluten-free diet (especially avoiding wheat) that still has some complex carbohydrates from brown rice, sweet potatoes, and legumes can give you a significant benefit.

CHAPTER SUMMARY

- The food you eat is critical to your cellular health and the health of your bodily systems.

- We can set general guidelines, but all PECs must get advice and tailor their diets to their particular challenges. Diets may need to change as PECs progress towards good health.

- Vegetarians and vegans must seek professional advice and be careful to follow the guidelines presented, as cutting out further foods may be detrimental. They may need to consider adjusting what they're willing to eat during recovery.

- It is essential to stop hypoglycaemic episodes that trigger the ANS dysfunction.

- The five pillars of the CFS recovery diet are as follows:

  1. Avoid foods and drinks that lead to blood glucose surges.

     – Eat only small amounts of sweet fruits.

     – Eat only small amounts of starchy carbohydrates and avoid refined starchy carbohydrates.

     – Avoid soft drinks and fruit juice.

  2. Avoid stimulants and toxins:

     – Avoid tea, coffee, and hot chocolate.

     – Avoid tobacco products.

     – Especially avoid alcohol.

     – Choose meat and seafood with fewer toxins.

     – Only eat the "dirty dozen" fruit and vegetables from organic sources

     – Avoid toxic oils, such as canola, cottonseed, corn, safflower, sunflower, and soybean oils.

     – Avoid trans fats by avoiding processed products and margarine.

     – Only cook with small amounts of stable fats like coconut oil and butter.

continued

3. Eat more vegetables, seeds, and nuts (although never peanuts and rarely pistachios and cashews).

4. Prepare food wisely. Prepare portions in advance, eat more raw foods, avoid microwaving, and wash and peel produce.

5. Eat regular, balanced meals. Make sure that your first and last meals of the day are well-balanced.

CHAPTER 18

Support with Supplements

An important note on supplementation!

Whilst most vitamins, minerals, and other supplements are generally safe, large amounts may have negative impacts on your health. You should always seek advice from an appropriately qualified person before starting a supplementation program.

The information in this book is for educational purposes only and is not to be taken as medical advice.

Before taking any supplements, you should check with your doctor and your pharmacist to make sure they are safe for you to take. This is especially true if you are taking medication. Even common vitamins and minerals can have unwanted effects when combined with some drugs.

Introduction to supplementation

Supplementing your food can have profound impacts on your health and recovery. Some of the changes will seem like a miracle.

Hundreds of supplements are available. Since you may have some level of dysfunction in virtually every aspect of your health, you may feel you should be taking every one of them. However, you need to use supplements wisely and with purpose.

To fully recover, you need to overcome the central and secondary illnesses of CFS, and taking supplements alone will normally not get you there.

However, getting the best nutrition possible can give you excellent results as part of your overall recovery program. This nutritional treatment, using food and supplements, is called orthomolecular medicine.

The term 'orthomolecular' was coined by Dr Linus Pauling, the only person to date to win two unshared Nobel prizes, one for chemistry and one for peace. Dr Pauling believed strongly in the power of nutrition and supplementation in treating a large range of diseases. A great deal of evidence shows the benefits of vitamin and mineral supplementation, and we've seen a growing movement towards integrative medicine.

If you have been sick for a long time and have seen alternative health practitioners, then you have probably tried taking large amounts of supplements with varied benefit. You might feel that all you have created is expensive urine.

However, as an analogy, just because you exercised once and it didn't get you the outcome you hoped for, doesn't mean that exercise is no good. And just because you took medicine once that didn't have the desired effect, didn't mean that you never tried any type of medicine again. Orthomolecular medicine can have an amazing restorative force when used scientifically and with focus.

Some supplementation guidelines

Here are some guidelines for better outcomes with supplementation.

Safety first

Do not assume that a substance is safe because it is 'natural', sold in large quantities to the general public, or used by other PECs. This is especially true if you are considering taking megadoses. It is important that you have a level-headed and balanced view of supplementation. Desperation can lead to foolhardy action, which can lead to negative consequences.

Few things are totally without risk and modern medicine is yet another example. There are inherent risks with taking any medication, having surgery or other medical treatments.

This might seem like an argument for doing nothing, but inaction can be disastrous as well. **My point is that anything that stops you from regaining your health is in fact doing you harm.**

Severe negative consequences caused by supplements are extremely rare and most often caused by contaminated product. But we are also concerned about other kinds of harm, so it's important to think through your supplementation plans.

Drugs and supplements can interact or 'double up'. For example, many people take blood thinning drugs. They may also want to take vitamin C or E, which are both natural blood-thinning agents. If they don't consider the doubling-up effect of taking the supplements along with the drug, and if they take extreme amounts, the impacts could be negative. So let me repeat myself: **If you are taking medication, you must seek advice from your doctor and pharmacist to ensure that you are not taking an undue risk.**

Remember, the body is amazingly complex, beyond anyone's current comprehension. Supplementation may have a positive impact, but especially when your body is dysfunctional, you should also consider any potential negative impacts, as in these examples:

- You might be able to immediately and drastically raise your detoxification, but are your liver and kidneys up to the job of getting rid of the products that will flood your bloodstream?

- You may be able to quickly rebuild your adrenal glands, but what impact will this have when your dysfunctional ANS floods your system with much higher levels of adrenal hormones?

Under normal circumstances in nature, vitamins and minerals are consumed as part of your food. Animals instinctively change their diet to make up imbalances or shortfalls. Getting minerals through foods ensures that they are bio-available and in appropriate amounts to sustain your body.

However, supplements may offer a vitamin or mineral in a form not found in nature or further down your body's biological processing line. Whilst skipping some processing can circumvent your body's biochemical dysfunctions, it can also be dangerous.

Here are a few examples of where more care needs to be taken in making decisions:

- A particularly active form of vitamin B12 is methylcobalamin. B12 is of interest to PECs for several reasons. If methylation is low, taking B12 supplements may help increase methylation and restore essential processes in the body. Methylcobalamin may be particularly useful if a PEC lacks certain enzymes. However, large amounts of it may be dangerous, as this molecule is an excellent heavy-metal detoxifier and can bind with mercury. Toxic build-up can be a real problem for PECs, and this adds the potential problem of having mercury fuse to methylcobalamin, which can cross the blood–brain barrier. It could take mercury from a biologically less active site (fat tissue, for example) and deposit it in a highly active site, such as neural tissue in the brain. But the most common form of B12, cyanocobalamin, usually doesn't exist in nature and is not directly used in the body. I believe that taking large amounts could cause problems for some PECs because of their dysfunctional biochemistry and their potential inability to process the cyanide in cyanocobalamin.

- Another supplement, called 5-Hydroxytryptophan (5-HTP), helps produce the neurotransmitters serotonin and melatonin. These neurotransmitters are often low in PECs, which interferes with their mood and sleep, so supplementation to support their production makes sense. This is especially true for people with poor gut function or for vegetarians or vegans who may not be getting enough of the essential amino acid tryptophan.

But this molecule is much further down the biosynthesis chain than natural food. Taking it to boost neurotransmitter production may have unintended consequences, especially if you are taking medication, in particular medication such as Prozac. Even if you are not, the 5-HTP is normally converted into serotonin in your nervous tissue and other tissues, such as your liver, kidneys, and intestines. Whilst boosting the serotonin and melatonin levels in your nervous tissue may be desirable, having high levels in your blood may lead to serious problems. In Germany, these are considered serious enough to make 5-HTP available only by prescription. Also, doctors in Germany often consider further medication to reduce the conversion of 5-HTP into serotonin outside of the nervous tissue.

Does this mean you should not take 5-HTP? Not necessarily, because it could help you over one of your hurdles. But you should definitely consider your decision carefully and seek professional advice.

- Fish oil may reduce inflammation (a major problem in CFS), but will taking twenty capsules a day cure CFS? Clearly not. Is it natural? No. Is it safe? That may depend on the manufacturer. How are the oils processed? Are they fresh or have they gone rancid? Does the product contain mercury? (You may want to consider krill oil as an alternative.) What other unintended consequences might supplementing at high levels have? How would it affect your lipid profile or your cholesterol production? If you want to change your omega-6 to omega-3 ratios from the common 20:1 or 30:1 to, say, 3:1, perhaps lowering your omega-6 consumption makes more sense.

Again, this doesn't mean you should do nothing. However, you should consider supplementation carefully.

I believe the most prudent approach is to be conservative but proactive. Get appropriate advice. Take supplements in small amounts, under medical supervision. Do your own homework and ask questions before accepting advice that seems unusual. **Remember, unusual does not mean wrong, and usual does not necessarily mean right.**

Be clear about your aims

A healthy person who has a good diet needs little supplementation to feel strong and healthy. (We might need some minerals to top up what's missing in modern fruits and vegetables.) PECs, however, can benefit from many supplements. But first you must ask yourself how effective they are and what their purpose is.

It makes sense to restore bodily and biochemical functions and to replenish nutrients lost over the years, rather than just plugging in an end product that your body is short of. Here's an example:

The coenzyme Q10 (CoQ10) is essential for many processes, most notably to create ATP for energy. What do you want from supplementing with this important vitamin-like substance? How long can you pay for it? Does the supplement actually fix the problem or just relieve it? If you use it primarily as an antioxidant, is there a better and cheaper alternative? Surely a better approach is to support your body so that it can make its own CoQ10 again, by giving it the building blocks—folic acid, vitamins B6, B12, B3, B5 and C, and the relevant trace elements. Perhaps most importantly, you'll also want to get your methylation cycle working to supply the methyl groups. Once methylation is functioning again, normal vitamin levels are restored, and your oxidative load has been reduced, you should have plenty of CoQ10. (This may not be true if you are taking a statin medication to lower your cholesterol.)

Supplementation makes good sense if you can afford it, and if your aim is to supplement for a period of time to reduce your symptoms. For example, after you've taken the CoQ10 for awhile, your nutrient levels and biochemical processes may be restored enough to reduce your symptoms. This will help you normalise your ANS more easily.

The real point here is to **have a plan** and not just take supplements to give you temporary relief without making any real lasting change in your body. **The aim should always be rebuilding your body to normal functioning, not covering up dysfunction.**

You can, of course, continue to take some supplements for the rest of your life.

Buy the best-quality supplements

The supplement industry is huge and growing fast. In the US alone, it was estimated to be worth around $26.9 billion in 2009 and it is still growing. The industry is regulated, but the products are not all tested and the actual quantities of the compounds often vary greatly from the description.

What is more important is the quality of the product. I am not talking about differences in quality between producers, but rather about the quality of the ingredients on the label.

For example, cheaper forms of magnesium, like the inorganic magnesium oxide, are more likely to give you loose stools than to increase your intracellular magnesium levels. A higher-quality product like magnesium citrate will offer better absorption. If your budget allows, a form chelated with amino acids is the best option.

As you recover, you may be better able to use poorer-quality supplements, but my advice is to always consider the quality. Buying something cheap that does not work is a waste of money. If you can be reasonably sure of the outcome, a few hundred dollars is a small price to pay for a significant and possibly life-changing impact.

Quality supplements may include the cofactors and coenzymes that make the supplement work. These are molecules that help with the biochemical transformation, so your body can make use of the supplement. They can include non-protein chemical compounds and metal ions such as manganese, cobalt, nickel, copper, zinc, and molybdenum. For example, when you are buying vitamin C, are you getting the bioflavonoids that help your body use the vitamin C? With most vitamin C supplements, you probably are not.

Choosing the right supplement is critical. Do you want to treat an imbalance or just increase levels? If you are treating an imbalance, using the mineral on its own may be appropriate. If you want to increase levels, you need to supply balancing minerals in the right proportion. If you are taking calcium, are you getting the right proportion of magnesium to balance it? The same applies to many other pairs of key minerals, such as sodium and potassium.

You also need to take the right amounts. You might think you're getting enough vitamin B5 because you take a B complex formula, but 50 mg won't do you much good if you need 1500 mg. (This is an example, not a recommendation.) With some supplements, you might get too much vitamin A or E, or even too much of a mineral such as iron. These can have negative effects. Most supplements have multiple ingredients. Even though you're not likely to end up with too much, it's still important to be diligent and add up the ingredients of everything you're taking. **I recommend you get advice from a health care professional rather than doing this by yourself.**

As I've said, taking a supplement that is not very bioavailable or does not have the required supporting cofactors will not be effective. If you are clear about what you intend to do, you are more likely to obtain the right product. You may want to buy supplements from a health care professional who can give you advice rather than just shopping for a deal online. Supplements that are cheap but ineffective become expensive.

Wean yourself off your supplements slowly

As with drugs, the body will adapt to certain nutrient intakes. If you don't reduce these gradually, you can have adverse outcomes.

Any herbs or other compounds such as adrenal cortex extracts (ACE), which affect the endocrine system directly or indirectly, need to be considered carefully. Suddenly stopping them may not leave your body enough time to adjust. Most of these compounds include hormones, but even if they don't, reducing them gradually will minimise a 'crash' effect. In my opinion, ACE products should not be taken at all unless all hormones have been removed. (See the next section for a more detailed discussion of ACEs.)

Another often-mentioned example is vitamin C. Some people say that if you take large amounts of vitamin C, then stop abruptly, you will get symptoms of scurvy or vitamin C deficiency. I believe this 'rebound scurvy' effect is a myth. Many doctors around the world now use megadose intravenous vitamin C therapy to help treat cancer without any such problems. However, PECs are much more sensitive to withdrawing such supports, so it's better to be cautious.

Get advice

You have probably already gathered that I think you should get advice rather than going it all alone. Don't imagine that you're an expert because you have read lots of conflicting information or because you have spent a small fortune on supplements. Experience may be more important than research. An experienced doctor or naturopath may have noted a difference in efficacy between two products that essentially claim to be the same.

The key is to get good advice. You need to know enough to differentiate good from bad.

Key areas for PECs to supplement

It is not practical for me to give information on every supplement that PECs may use. This would overwhelm you with information that may or may not be relevant to you.

But here are several critical areas which merit further detail:

Mineral replenishment and balancing

For many PECs, this will be the first issue to be addressed. Some naturopaths use hair mineral analysis to gauge deficiencies and imbalances. Whilst such tests may be insightful, their accuracy is questionable and hence should not be relied on in isolation.

Magnesium supplementation must be a first consideration for PECs. Not only is it involved in countless bodily functions, it is also central to producing energy. Significant magnesium supplementation can have drastic effects on energy levels, stiffness, and general wellbeing, and produce better cellular and detoxification functions. Different sources recommend different amounts for PECs, from 200 to 700 mg. My suggestion is that you continue to take some magnesium to maintain your magnesium levels even after you have recovered.

As your magnesium stores are replenished and you feel better, you may also add some calcium, to maintain your calcium/magnesium ratio. However, be careful with calcium as it may make fibromyalgia symptoms worse. Getting calcium from food is usually preferable.

The other key mineral is sodium. We live in a salt-phobic world, mainly due to fear campaigns about excessive salt in processed foods, and because of and the link to hypertension. Let's be clear: Excessive salt is bad, as is hypertension. However, if you follow my diet guidelines, you will be eating far fewer processed foods, eliminating these high levels of sodium. You then need to replace this with the healthier option of quality sea salt without additives.

But in many cases, the problem is not sodium consumption but the way it is regulated by the adrenal glands. PECs who have been ill for a long time are likely to have adrenal insufficiency. They will lose sodium as the body produces less of the hormone aldosterone. This can lead to an imbalance between sodium and potassium, which is critical to maintaining cellular health and good blood pressure.

If your sodium levels are depleted, it is important to restore your reserves to healthy levels. Low blood pressure and inability to maintain blood pressure (dizziness) as you rise from a lying position can be signs of inadequate sodium levels. So are salt cravings, which you may have experienced.

However, given that some PECs have exactly the opposite problems, especially early on in their illness or during some exacerbations, you need to ensure that your blood pressure does not rise to unacceptable levels. **If you have hypertension problems, you do not need to increase your blood pressure. Increasing salt intake in such cases could be dangerous. Speak with your doctor.**

Also, be sure to drink enough quality water (without poisons such as chlorine or fluoride, where possible) to improve your hydration. If you have excessive thirst due to depleted sodium levels, drinking more may exacerbate the problem. It may wash more salt out of your system and cause you to lose potassium. However, taking potassium is not generally recommended. You should have enough potassium if you eat significantly more fresh fruits and vegetables.

Energy production

A large number of supplements are used in the production of ATP. These include magnesium and the B vitamins (B1, B2, B3, B5, B6 B7, B9, and B12), as well as malic acid, coenzyme Q10, and the sugar D-ribose. Recommended amounts vary. Table 3 shows ranges of amounts recommended for PECs by doctors, researchers, and commentators.

Supplements alone will not fix your energy crisis, but they will help generate ATP. Restoring your reserves of essential nutrients is critical. Perhaps magnesium has the most important role here.

In my opinion, as your energy levels improve, you might taper off coenzyme Q10, D-ribose, and malic acid, then reduce the B vitamins to a more normal level (like the recommended daily amount). You might want to continue supplementing magnesium and vitamin B12 (cyanocobalamin or hydroxocobalamine), at perhaps half the levels recommended in the table below.

Once again, talk to your healthcare professional for personalised recommendations.

Supplement	Lower Range	Upper Range
B1 (thiamine)	25 mg	75 mg
B2 (riboflavin)	25 mg	75 mg
B3 (niacin or niacinamide)	25 mg	125 mg
B5 (pantothenic acid)	50 mg	1500 mg
B6 (pyridoxine, etc.)	25 mg	100 mg
B7 (biotin)	150 mcg	200 mcg
B9 (folic acid)	400 mcg	800 mcg
B12 (various cobalamines)	50 mcg	1000 mcg
Magnesium	200 mg	700 mg
Coenzyme Q10 (CoQ10)	100 mg	200 mg
Malic acid	500 mg	1500 mg
D-ribose	10 g	15 g

Table 3 : Range Of Recommendations (by various commentators) for Energy Supplementation

Adrenal recovery

Most PECs are likely to have some level of adrenal insufficiency, particularly if they have been sick for longer than one or two years. In fact, for many PECs, this condition may get quite extreme.

Treating adrenal insufficiency may not be a good idea until the ANS dysfunction has been addressed. The ability to produce more adrenal hormones may be detrimental, as it can exacerbate cortisol surges. Also, the lack of adrenal hormones may be more due to a regulation problem than an inability to produce them.

Hence I favour allowing the adrenals to restore themselves naturally, as the ANS function normalises. The changes to exercise, stress management and diet described in this book will go far towards helping your adrenals recover.

However, supplementation is also very important to ensure that the required materials are available to rebuild the adrenals. Whilst the energy supplements also support adrenal recovery, various other supplements need to be considered more carefully.

Let me start with one that is not controversial, vitamin C.

Vitamin C

Vitamin C is very important in the rebuilding of adrenals. Reasonably large amounts of vitamin C are useful. Different practitioners recommend different amounts—from 1-4 g per day, but sometimes much higher levels. Strong vitamin C therapy has other benefits, chiefly stimulating your immune system. This vitamin should definitely be used by every PEC. You need to buy a quality product that includes bioflavonoids.

Hydrocortisone

Perhaps the most contentious substance used in adrenal recovery is hydrocortisone. This drug is the artificial version of cortisol. The theory is that, whilst you take this, your adrenals don't have to produce cortisol and can replenish their hormonal stores. Whilst small amounts may have shown some therapeutic effect, I believe that we are interfering with the natural feedback regulation of cortisol in the body. I also believe you must taper off this medication extremely slowly, even when you have been taking only small amounts, or it may leave you feeling worse than before.

In some extreme cases, small therapeutic amounts of 20 mg or less may be called for, but they must only be taken under the eye of a very experienced medical doctor. **My personal preference is to avoid hydrocortisone therapy where possible.** Correcting the ANS dysfunction and providing supplements for energy production is a better strategy for most PECs, in my view.

Adrenal cortex extract (ACE)

It's my view that a potentially better alternative to hydrocortisone is adrenal cortex extract (ACE), which is obtained from the adrenal glands of cattle and other domestic food animals. These products were in widespread use until pharmaceutical companies invented hydrocortisone. Since then, the use of ACE has been much reduced and even outlawed in some places. The benefit of the natural product is that it contains substances to rebuild the adrenal glands. However, these products can still contain hormones. Whilst they are natural, they may still interfere with your own hormone regulation. Reducing your dosage needs to be done very gradually as well. Products that do not contain hormones may have fewer withdrawal side effects.

I believe ACEs can be very helpful if taken in significant amounts. However, in my opinion, the ACE must be of good quality and should not contain hormones. Such products are hard to find, but they do exist. Make sure that you get advice from a professional when choosing a product and double check that the product is legal to import in your part of the world, before making any purchases.

Herbs for adrenal recovery

I will not discuss herbs in detail here. If you are interested in them, I recommend that you do your research thoroughly. My concern is that the mechanism of how herbs function is not always fully understood. Many of them stimulate or replace hormonal functions. Whilst this may have a good effect in the short term, it may also have an impact on your own feedback cycles and possibly interrupt longer-term hormone regulation. This is already a problem for PECs, so you should do nothing that could make this worse. **I recommend you be conservative with herbs.**

Methylation support and detoxification

I believe that problems with detoxification are a key problem in many PECs. As I discussed earlier, Dr Konyenburg proposed a glutathione depletion theory as the cause of CFS. In my opinion, his explanation of the pathophysiology is very good. However, I believe that ANS dysfunction is the central cause of CFS and that methylation issues are secondary.

The methylation problems he proposes usually include genetic variations, such as the MTHFR mutation, making many people worry that something is broken in them. But I want to remind people that many PECs do not have that mutation, and that other people who do have it, often live perfectly healthy lives. Further, I believe that this may not even be the most relevant enzyme in methylation, but that it has been talked about because it is easier to test. So investigating this in too much detail and having expensive gene tests done may simply be a distraction from the real problem.

Still, supporting methylation and glutathione production may be helpful to many PECs. The question is how this is best achieved and how much to intervene or support it.

Methylation protocol

Whilst glutathione levels are fairly consistently low in PECs, methylation is not necessarily so. Whilst **some PECs clearly show signs of hypomethylation (under-methylation),** others do not. It has also been suggested that some PECs, especially those with MCS, may **show signs of hypermethylation (over-methylation).** I am not convinced that this is an accurate interpretation of the data or that such a state of hypermethlation actually exists. However, if it does, then orthomolecular support to boost methylation further would clearly not be a good idea.

So whilst methylation may be an important part of the problems of CFS, you need to be certain about your actual methylation status.

One fairly strong indicator for hypomethylation is elevated histamine and/or basophiles. However, these tests may not be conclusive, so they should not be the only thing you rely on. The guidance of an experienced doctor is very important. Such a doctor may specialise in treating autism using the Yasko protocol or have an association with the Walsh Institute. However, these are different schools of thought and they may have differences of opinion about treatment, since this area of science is still not well established.

I feel that, as with adrenal insufficiency, the normalising of the ANS dysfunction will reduce pressure on glutathione and methylation. As your health improves, adequate function should return.

But some people may need help to experience adequate methylation, especially if they have been unwell for a long period of time. But before even considering this, I think it is most important to

confirm whether you have a problem with methylation and what that problem is.

If we know, or strongly suspect, that a PEC has unusual methylation, **only then treatment may be appropriate.** However, opinions vary as to what promotes methylation and what depresses it. For example, some biochemists and researchers believe that folate supplements suppress methylation and some believe they promote it.

The important point is that **if experts can't agree, then how can you confidently follow any such treatment program?**

Hence I recommend that PECs tread very carefully when considering supplements for methylation. This is an extremely complicated area of science, one that is not yet fully understood. What works best for an individual depends upon their particular methylation status and genetic make-up. You should therefore only treat this problem with supplements after you know for certain that over- or under-methylation is actually occurring.

A simplified methylation protocol is available on the Internet, but I have not included it here because **I don't believe that PECs should proceed with such a treatment without the supervision and guidance of an experienced doctor.**

Tests continue to grow in this specialised area of medicine. You may want to consider tests that accurately determine where the actual (not theoretical) bottleneck or poor functioning is occurring before embarking on a treatment program. The key is to find a doctor to interpret the results, one who will not have you spend thousands of dollars on unnecessary supplements. I understand that finding such a doctor may be very difficult and that this type of testing may be outside of your budget. In my view, this whole area of treatment should be considered as supportive, not critical for the vast majority of people.

Other detoxification support

The vitamins and minerals previously mentioned will also support the liver in detoxification.

However, it is also important to have adequate amino acids, notably glutamine, glycine, taurine, and cysteine. You may also supplement antioxidants such as vitamin E, together with zinc and a number of herbs, including St. Mary's thistle (milk thistle), globe artichoke, slippery elm bark, and dandelion.

You may not need this additional support as your body starts functioning more normally again. I have listed these for more stubborn liver conditions.

As always, you should be guided by your doctor or naturopath who can recommend a 'liver tonic' that fits your needs as part of an overall program. Given the overlap in vitamin B supplements, a comprehensive treatment program is better than an ad-hoc, shotgun approach.

Neurotransmitter support

In my book *Discover Hope*, I discuss depression and the challenges of coping with CFS. Several neurotransmitters are implicated in depression, chiefly **serotonin, norepinephrine,** and **dopamine**.

Several classes of antidepressants affect these *and other* neurotransmitters. The impact of medication on biochemistry and the interaction with drugs and other supplements becomes complex, as can withdrawal from such drugs. **This is another reason to be under medical advice.**

But depression isn't the only impact of neurotransmitter imbalances. They can affect a variety of different mental conditions, including anxiety, schizophrenia, obsessive–compulsive disorder, and even general mental functioning.

Whilst an in-depth discussion of this is beyond the scope of this book, I will make a few observations, which may suggest the use of other supplements. However, the biochemistry of neurotransmitters is complicated. We can't simply say, "You are missing X, so take X," or "Take an X-uptake inhibitor."

A good starting point is the common dysfunctions in PECs. The chief one is the imbalance of the ANS, which affects many different biochemical processes. The main dysfunction is the excessive (and, at times, insufficient) release of adrenalin and norepinephrine (noradrenalin). So just providing support (or uptake inhibitors) for these neurotransmitters won't fix everything. The central cause of CFS must be addressed in conjunction with other treatments for a real long-term solution.

But other neurotransmitters are also implicated. A breakdown in methylation can affect these neurotransmitters, hence the studies in methylation support for depression. Methylation is directly involved in converting serotonin to melatonin, producing epinephrine and acetylcholine, as well as eliminating dopamine.

Methylation is critical in producing choline, which is used to make acetylcholine. Since acetylcholine is critical for arousal and smooth brain functioning, a reduction in methylation may contribute to the 'brain fog' symptoms of CFS.

So what does this all mean in terms of supplementation? I would suggest, first and foremost, that you recover from CFS and normalise your biochemical functions. However, assisting the normalisation of your neurotransmitters will greatly help your recovery by improving functioning. Let's look at the various way you can do this.

Amino acids

Two amino acids are of particular interest, tryptophan and tyrosine.

Tryptophan is converted into 5-HTP, which is used to make serotonin, which in turn is used to make melatonin, which is critical to sleep. Different doctors and researchers suggest supplementing 5-HTP with 100 mg to 300 mg per day. If you pursue this, I would suggest starting conservatively under medical supervision. **In my experience, the benefits of this supplementation can be significant.**

Tyrosine is the building block for dopamine, which is used to make norepinephrine and epinephrine. If these neurotransmitters are low, tyrosine supplements may benefit you. However, keep in mind that this biochemical pathway is central to the dysfunctions of CFS. Whilst supplementation may be very beneficial for normally-depressed people, it might exacerbate PECs' conditions. **I would approach tyrosine supplementation with great caution**, and, if you do consider it, preferably defer it until you are significantly recovered.

Herbs

The best known herb for depression is St. John's wort. However, just because it is natural doesn't mean it doesn't warrant respect. We do not understand the precise mechanism of how it works, but its efficacy is well known. You should definitely consider it if you are suffering severe symptoms of depression, but you must seek medical advice first. In particular, double check with your MD and pharmacist if you are on any medications, in particular SSRIs or other neurogenic drugs.

Zinc

PECs are often very low in zinc. It has a wide range of benefits for immune function, DNA function, and gene expression. It also plays a role in brain function and could even be considered as a neurotransmitter.

However, zinc is a double-edged sword, as too much zinc can be a problem and possibly act as a neurotoxin. Whilst small amounts of zinc are probably fine as part of your multivitamin and mineral support, therapeutic dosages should only be used under medical supervision. Your doctor should monitor blood levels for zinc and possibly consider hair mineral analysis. (Hair analysis is less accurate, but it may give some indication of zinc levels.)

Other vitamins and minerals

Neurotransmitter production is greatly assisted by the B vitamins and vitamin C. Magnesium, manganese, copper, and iron act as catalysts.

Closing words on neurotransmitter supplementation

Rebuilding neurotransmitters with supplements can be an extremely powerful way to start feeling better. However, blindly adding these nutrients without deeper consideration is not a good idea. Also, long-term use may not be appropriate.

If you are taking antidepressant medication, some of these supplements may be dangerous. Similarly, other medication, especially blood thinners or oral contraception, may not be compatible with your supplements. You should therefore seek advice, ideally from a holistic doctor, to explore supplementation options.

The importance of vitamin D

Vitamin D is an important nutrient/hormone for good health. It aids immune function and protects against a range of chronic diseases, such as cancer and heart disease. It is difficult to get vitamin D from food, and supplements are not a good alternative as the vitamin may not be readily converted into a sulphate version. The best way to get vitamin D is to get sun exposure. We are all aware of the risk of skin cancer, so excess exposure is not a good idea. However, some daily exposure on large parts of your body (not just your arms and hands) will help you get an adequate amount of this important pro-hormone. Don't wash your vitamin D down the drain by showering immediately after sun exposure; give your skin some time to absorb it.

Important final words on supplementation

A big trap for PECs is seeing supplementation and orthomolecular medicine as the cure for CFS, and getting more and more involved in the complex world of biochemistry and physiology. Instead of trying to 'fix the body', I believe a better approach is to focus on normalising the ANS dysfunction, correcting diet and exercise, and then using 'supportive supplementation' to help the body to heal and return to normal functioning.

The difference is subtle but important. 'Fixing the body' means adding compounds to correct different dysfunctions. 'Supportive supplementation' means realising that the body knows best how to correct its functions, but we give it help or fuel to get the job done.

Too much focus on or concern about symptoms, trying to 'fix biochemical dysfunctions', or 'finding a cure' for CFS is likely to perpetuate the ANS dysfunction and delay recovery. It seems most reasonable to **focus first on correcting the ANS dysfunction, restoring gut function, and correcting mineral deficiencies and mitochondrial dysfunction**. I expect that this approach plus a supportive diet will lead to recovery for the vast majority of PECs.

In my opinion, if you've been diagnosed with adrenal insufficiency or methylation problems, you should consider supervised supplementation only after some time and significant recovery (around 65–90%). But you must be sure that your recovery has plateaued because of these problems and not because of an inability to shift your focus from your symptoms or other sources of stress. This is obviously difficult to evaluate, so careful analysis is required.

CHAPTER SUMMARY

- Use supplements wisely and with purpose.

- Make sure that your supplementation is safe, and get professional advice on specific products.

- Take a conservative but proactive approach to supplementation to avoid complications.

- Do your own research and ask questions of your health care adviser.

- Be clear about your intentions for supplementation. Aim to rebuild your body's functions, not cover up dysfunctions.

- Buy only high-quality supplements with high bioavailability.

- Wean yourself off supplements slowly.

- Get professional advice.

- Take a comprehensive approach to mineral supplementation.

- Consider starting with more comprehensive energy-reaction supplements, then taper off to only a few supplements, at lower doses.

- Only consider adrenal recovery and hypomethylation treatments if recovery of these dysfunctions has definitely plateaued.

- Consider hydrocortisone and adrenal cortex extracts very carefully, if at all, and only under medical supervision. Be careful to reduce such medication and supplementation very gradually.

- Supplement with quality vitamin C, for adrenal recovery and to build your immune functions.

- Ensure that you have researched herbs very carefully, especially ones that affect endocrine function.

- Only consider a methylation protocol under experienced medical supervision, as adverse reactions have been noted.

- Be careful not to get too focused on treatments, as your ANS may interpret this as concern and go back on high alert.

CHAPTER 19

Exercise

"I have never taken any exercise except sleeping and resting."

- Mark Twain

Is exercise your enemy or your friend? This can be a topic of great controversy for PECs, and for good reason.

The standard recommendation from doctors is **Graded Exercise Therapy (GET),** that is, slowly increasing exercise over time.

However, if you are like many people, you have probably found that even if you increase your exercise very slowly, eventually you experience a crash. So your past experience with exercise may have put you off.

Since the primary cause of CFS is not a lack of exercise, exercise alone isn't likely to fix anything. But the human body and endocrine system were not designed for the sedentary lifestyle that PECs experience or the large quantities of carbohydrates that we typically consume.

Exercise, like nutrition, is a complicated topic and a wide range of hotly-contested opinions. I ask you to put any preconceptions on hold for a moment and consider what I say with an open mind. (Note that some of my definitions in this text may vary slightly from the general definitions and some biological processes are simplified.)

First, let's explore types of exercise and their impact on the body.

Types of exercise

Broadly speaking, you can divide exercise into three categories:

- Flexibility and lymphasising activities: Stretching, deep breathing, and slow and gentle movements that lead to lengthened muscles and the movement of lymphatic fluid to supply new nutrients and remove waste products.
- Strength training: The use of resistance to work muscles to build strength and anaerobic endurance.
- Endurance training: The use of repetitive movement over a longer period of time to build endurance by increasing the capacity of the cardiovascular system and cellular functions.

Exercise can also be classified according to its intensity and how it forces the body into different cellular respiration to create energy:

- Very light aerobic exercise: Activity that does not cause the person doing the exercise to notice an increase in heart rate.
- Low-intensity aerobic exercise: Activity that raises the heart rate comfortably, without strain, and does not force glucose metabolism. (more about this later)
- High-intensity aerobic exercise: Activity that raises the heart rate, creates significant discomfort, and does force glucose metabolism.
- Very-high-intensity anaerobic exercise: Activity with enough intensity to force a switch to anaerobic glucose metabolism, where lactic acid is created.

The purpose of exercise for PECs

Despite their difficulties with exercise, PECs can benefit for a number of reasons.

- It's good to stimulate lymph fluid to flow throughout your tissues. It ensures that your cells have adequate nutrition and that harmful waste products don't pool and create cellular dysfunction. Instead, your body can mobilise toxins for processing in appropriate ways.

- Exercise has a positive effect on mood. It can thus assist in reducing stress and normalising the ANS dysfunction. Over time, PECs can regain confidence in their ability to be active and can stop monitoring their bodies for symptoms.
- Exercise can reduce insulin resistance and, together with diet, can encourage fatty acid metabolism and normal blood sugar regulation. This lowers hypoglycaemic cortisol responses that sensitise the ANS.
- Exercise rehabilitates the body so that PECs recover the strength and endurance to take part in normal, healthy life activities without excessive physical stress. So it reduces the impact of physical activity and reduces the possibility of relapse.

As you can see, exercise provides important benefits, besides the fact that it can be enjoyable. Yet many PECs seem to crash every time they build up their exercise levels. This takes them back to square one in their recovery and leaves them feeling more discouraged than ever.

Why?

The answer, as always, is in the details.

Understanding your energy envelope

Exercise can oxygenate our tissues and release endorphins, giving us the 'exercise high' that is so addictive—or it can flood our tissues with acid and cortisol in response to severe stress. How do you do the former and avoid the latter?

To really understand exercise, you may want to reread the discussion about the energy metabolism pathways in Part Two of the book.

As you might remember, when the body has an excessive demand for energy, ATP is still converted to ADP, but ADP is also converted to AMP, which is lost via urine. **This means that if you exercise too hard or too long, you will exceed your capacity to create cellular energy. This energy crisis will cause secondary problems that perpetuate CFS. You must avoid this at all costs.**

Do not push yourself. We are often conditioned to believe that we should push through or soldier on through fatigue. But resting when you are tired is essential, or you will exacerbate your problems.

PECs usually start to exercise gently; then, as they start to feel better because more oxygen is available (for more energy) and as lymph fluid becomes more mobile (for more energy and to remove toxins), they start to feel more confident and try to do more. Up to this point, the process sounds pretty similar to GET. The problem for PECs is that they then increase their activity beyond their 'energy envelope'. This pushes them into a toxic mode of energy creation, which depresses the immune system, acidifies tissues, and increases stress hormones.

Whilst a healthy person can deal much better with increases in stress, acidity, and immune dysfunction, a PEC is thrown back into the dysfunction cycles of CFS.

Before we can understand the conditions that allow PECs to exercise wisely, we have to understand a little more physiology.

Burning glucose, fat, or glucose from fat and protein

Yes, this is a confusing topic, and an area of some disagreement. As before, for simplicity's sake, I will ignore certain energy pathways.

In the section on mitochondrial dysfunction, we looked at aerobic and anaerobic metabolism and the difference in the amount of energy created. (The aerobic type creates much more energy.) But energy is created in a much more complex way, depending on many factors.

This is because carbohydrates are not the only nutrient used to create energy. Protein and fat can also be used in several different pathways. Protein and fat get mobilised and broken down during a glucose crisis (low blood sugar state) and are used in the Krebs cycle to create ATP.

So what determines whether, glucose, fat, or protein is used to create energy?

Protein is only broken down for energy during a crisis when cortisol is released. We want to avoid this pathway if we are to rebuild muscle tissue and reduce insulin resistance. Also, I believe the excessive, chronic breakdown of proteins leads to pressure on your biochemistry and to secondary problems such as mitochondrial dysfunction.

The important point is whether you use fat or glucose for energy. These are the differences between using fats and carbohydrates:

- Only a relatively small amount of carbohydrates is available at any one time (compared to relatively large reserves of fat).
- A diet for direct fat metabolism does not create as much acid as one for carbohydrate metabolism.

However, unlike carbohydrates, which essentially have one pathway into the Krebs cycle, fatty acids can enter the Krebs cycle in two ways. First, they can be converted into glucose, primarily by your liver, then follow the usual glucose metabolism route and enter the cells with the help of insulin. Second, they can be used directly via a process called beta oxidation, where the fatty acids are absorbed into the cell and turned in acetyl-CoA for entry into the Krebs cycle.

The difference is that **the beta oxidation pathway does not affect your blood sugar levels. It can thus be thought of as a buffer for your energy requirements.** This is the energy your muscles normally use whilst at rest.

If you need more energy than beta oxidation can provide, then aerobic glucose metabolism takes over. If you have only a small supply of glucose, then both muscle fibres and the liver can provide more by breaking down fatty acids (and protein).

It is only when aerobic activity does not provide enough energy that the anaerobic metabolism of glycolysis takes over. This ultimately leads to lactic acid build-up. Aerobic activity is normally limited by the speed with which oxygen can diffuse into the muscles. However, I believe that in PECs it is also limited by the inefficiency of glucose transfer (due to insulin resistance) and due to mitochondrial depletion and dysfunction.

So back to our original question:

What determines whether glucose, fat, or protein is used to create energy?

We're getting technical now, so let's look at Figure 11 to help us understand this in more detail.

As you can see in Figure 11, fatty acids are burned in the Krebs cycle at rest and in low-intensity activity. As intensity increases, **aerobic** glucose metabolism takes over. Then your body switches to **anaerobic** glucose metabolism, creating lactic acid and an oxygen debt. This can only be sustained for shorter periods, say, 90 seconds.

During very intense exercise, once the available ATP in your cells is used up (say, after five seconds), you have another eight to ten seconds of energy from the phosphagen system. This is a minor system only used for very high-intensity exercise.

But if your fatty acid metabolism does not provide energy fast enough, and if you run out of glucose, your body will create glucose from fat and protein via a process called gluconeogenesis.

This breakdown in amino acids is trigged by cortisol. It burdens the system with ammonia, a toxic by-product that is usually excreted via urea. **An overload of ammonia can impair neurological functions and cause muscle fatigue.**

I believe that a much better mechanism is to condition your body to use fat directly via the beta oxidation pathway. This can only be done by exercising at lower intensities and increasing intensity only as you improve the mitochondrial function of fatty acid metabolism.

How exactly do you do this?

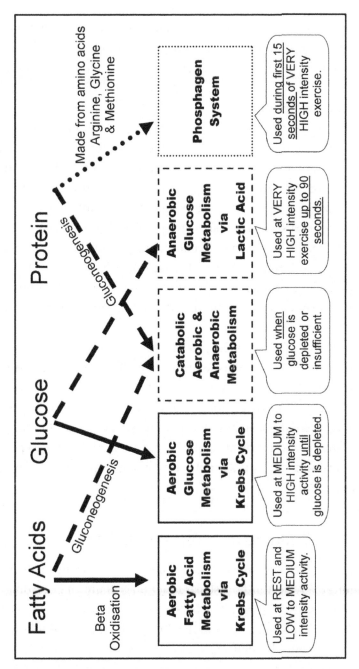

Figure 11: Simplified Intensity Mediated Energy Metabolism Pathways

I believe **you need increased numbers of well-functioning mitochondria and sufficient carnitine**. Carnitine is an amino acid found in animal products which can also be created by the body if methylation is functioning normally. It is used to transport fatty acids for use in the mitochondria.

Another important factor is **conditioning**. The human body is wonderful at adapting. I believe that you can improve your fatty acid respiration by somewhat **reducing your intake of carbohydrates** (especially grains and processed grain products) and **increasing the intake of quality fats,** whilst exercising daily at **low intensity**.

However, intense, prolonged exercise causes oxidative stress. That is the last thing a PEC wants. It puts more pressure on an already-struggling detoxification system and reduce glutathione levels; it is also likely to make mitochondrial dysfunction worse. **I believe that intense exercise is absolutely detrimental to PECs. You should avoid it until you have recovered.**

Interestingly enough, once you are fully recovered, some short **bursts of very high-intensity exercise** can have significant health benefits, given that they can increase your levels of growth hormone and testosterone. However, these should always be short, say, five bursts of 30 seconds, as opposed to chronic exercise like running for twenty minutes or more at a glucose-burning rate. **This type of interval training is not suitable for PECs, especially early in recovery.**

Building an exercise regimen

PECs who have been unwell for a long time have many challenges in resuming exercise. Cardiovascular function is diminished, leading to excessive intensity (measured by heart rate) at a low workload (say, a fast walk). Muscular strength and flexibility are diminished following long periods of muscle-reducing stress.

So if you quickly resume exercise, not only are you likely to overdo it, but you may also suffer injuries and inflammation that put further stress on the body and can cause a relapse. The important thing is not the size of your leg muscles or biceps but the condition of the smaller interconnecting muscles that support your overall structure.

The key is to proceed slowly.

Initial rehabilitation and yoga

An ideal exercise would be gentle and do the following:

- Reduce stress by making you breathe deeply, to reduce the arousal in your cortex and amygdalae.
- Promote the movement of lymphatic fluid and gently build up your interconnecting and main muscle groups to a stage that allows exercise beyond walking.

One such exercise is yoga. Here are its benefits on various bodily systems:

- Lymphatic system: The lymphatic system does not have an organ to move its fluid, the way the heart moves blood. It relies on the movement of the body. The inversion, twist, backbend, and other dynamic yoga poses promote the movement of lymphatic fluid to replenish tissues with nutrients and help carry away waste.
- Nervous system: The easing of muscle tension and the focusing of the mind on the breath and movements combine to calm the nervous system. Long-term benefits include reduced stress and anxiety levels.
- Cardiovascular system (heart and arteries): Regular yoga practise may help normalise blood pressure.
- Digestive system: Improved blood circulation and a massaging effect speed up digestion and help with undigested bowel matter.
- Musculoskeletal system: Maintaining poses promotes strength and endurance, whilst gentle stretching releases muscle tension and increases flexibility. Other benefits may include reduced back pain and improved posture. Also, joints move through their full range of motion, which encourages mobility.

Yoga is a great starting point, but make sure you practice with a skilled teacher. Do not try to do it on your own. Incorrect practice can cause injuries and other problems. It is important that PECs treat even the gentlest of classes with respect until their cardiovascular and adrenal systems normalise and their musculoskeletal system strengthens. The great thing about yoga is that it is a lifelong practice that never becomes too easy. As you improve, you can always increase its challenge.

An alternative to yoga may be tai chi or chi gong; however, I feel that yoga is preferable for most PECs.

'Cardio' exercise

We're actually looking for fat-burning exercises rather than cardiovascular exercises, but the most important thing is intensity. How do you know when an exercise is too intense? Experts have tried to set appropriate heart rates with convoluted formulas, but table 4 tries to summarise this for you.

I believe that PECs should initially aim to bring their heart rate to the bottom end of the aerobic fat-burning zone, at 60% of their maximum heart rate. You may be surprised how little you have to do to get to this rate. Walking may be your best exercise.

The best way to measure your heart rate is with a heart rate monitor that straps around your chest and sends a signal to a watch or to the equipment at a gym. But use it only as a guide.

Don't put all your focus on making sure you are in the 'right' range. Make sure that you enjoy the experience of exercising. Appreciate your surroundings and what you are doing, especially if you are exercising outdoors.

You should **limit your exercise time to twenty minutes,** with a ten-minute warm-up and a ten-minute cool-down. This 40 minutes may be too much for you initially. If so, begin by doing only the warm-up and cool-down routines described below. Build up to doing these for twenty minutes, then slowly add a bit of higher intensity exercise (at 60% of max rate), until you have built up to 40 minutes.

Age	60% of Max Rate		70% of Max Rate		80 % of Max Rate	Max (calc.) Heart Rate
15	123	☺	144	😐	164	205
20	120		140		160	200
25	117		137		156	195
30	114		133		152	190
35	111		130		148	185
40	108	Aerobic Fat Burning Zone	126	Cardio Endurance Building Zone	144	180
45	105		123		140	175
50	102		119		136	170
55	99		116		132	165
60	96		112		128	160
65	93		109		124	155
70	90		105		120	150
75	87		102		116	145
80	84	☺	98	😐	112	140
85	81		95		108	135

	↑		↑
	ideal start		upper limit

Table 4 : Fat Burning and Cardio Endurance Heart Rate Zones

Realise that warm-ups and cool-downs are absolutely critical and should be prioritised in your workout routine.

The essential warm-up

Don't fall into the trap of thinking that you are only exercising lightly and don't need a warm-up. In fact, 'warm-up' is the wrong term. I am not concerned about the level of heat in your muscles but about switching your metabolism on for fat burning.

In order to burn fat, you need to have the fat where it can be used. During your warm-up, your body mobilises your fat stores into fatty acids that are transported for use in your muscle cells.

This can be easiest to accomplish on a treadmill, using a heart-rate monitor. For the first five minutes, I focus on building up, very gradually, to walking at a pace halfway between my standing pulse and my target range. I maintain this rate until the last two minutes of the warm-up, and then increase at my own pace until I reach the target zone.

You don't have to be this exact. Just spend ten minutes walking at a very slow pace that is less than your target rate and ease slowly into your exercise. Slower is better.

The essential cool-down

After you have finished your twenty minutes of fat-burning exercise, you need to cool down for another ten minutes. The first five minutes will most likely be spent reducing your heart rate, leaving the last five minutes for walking at the reduced rate.

This is essential to ensure that the used blood with its toxins gets delivered to the appropriate places to be purified and reoxygenated. Failure to do so can leave your tissues exposed to the very toxic products that you are trying to get rid of.

When you finish your cool-down, spend five minutes relaxing your muscles and stretching them gently. Perform very gentle, dynamic breathing exercises by moving your arms slowly and bending and stretching. This should maximise movement of your lymph fluid.

Making adjustments

You need to listen to your body. Your senses are the best way to tell if you are moving out of your ideal fat-burning zone. If you start to mouth-breathe or huff and puff, or if you find that your eyesight is narrowing or your eyes or body are tensing, you are likely in sugar-burning mode and need to slow down.

Don't worry if you get to this point quickly. Once you recover from CFS, you can add some cardio training to improve your fitness. But during your recovery, build up only very gradually.

Whilst you can build up your exercise sessions to a heart rate 70% of maximum and a length of 50 minutes (including warm-up and cool-down), don't be tempted to do more than that. Also, for the first month, exercise only two or three times a week. Graduate to daily exercise only if it feels right.

If 40 minutes feels like too much, exercise for 30. If 30 minutes are too much, do twenty, or even just ten minutes. You get the idea. If you are not feeling up to exercising at all, then perhaps just take a five-minute stroll. Enjoy sitting in the park, relaxing and listening to the birds and breathing deeply, or have a meditation session with some gentle tai-chi-like movements to promote lymphasising.

Your progress is not measured by your performance, so relax and go with the flow. If you suddenly do feel like doing a lot more, pull back the reins. Whenever you are doing less than you can, you are helping to maintain or build up your reserves.

Your aim should be to feel great and reenergised at the end of every session. You should not feel depleted.

Weight training

I would not advise doing weight training until you have somewhat recovered. Most weight training is anaerobic, so it carries with it the potential to drive you into cortisol territory and set you back.

When most people train with weights, they push hard beyond what they are capable of. Pushing yourself hard with hyper-aroused ANS is not a good idea. This not only applies to your workout sessions, but also to your total weekly exercise regime.

If you have built up to comfortable daily walks without setbacks, drop back to two or three per week and add one and then two weight sessions per week.

For your weight training sessions, I recommend a ten-minute warm-up as usual and then five minutes of higher-intensity work to get some heat into your muscles. Don't overdo it, but if you can build up a light sweat, that would be great.

I believe the following workout guidelines work best for PECs:

- Stay focused on the goal—good health. You are not trying to break records or look like a body-building champ. You are trying to rebuild your muscles without triggering the excessive cortisol that will have a counterproductive effect, breaking down your muscles and increasing your CFS symptoms.

- Keep your workouts simple. Don't worry about writing down every little thing you are doing and building up your weights. Instead, use your instincts. If you can't do as much this week as you did last week, it doesn't matter. Listen to your body.

- I would suggest you limit your sets per exercise to one warm-up set of around fifteen to twenty repetitions followed by one or two sets of six to ten with a heavier weight.

- Keep your workouts short, **no more than fifteen minutes (plus warm-up and cool-down)**. So your sessions will consist of only two or three different exercises. An example might include the following areas:
    - Legs and calves
    - Back and biceps
    - Shoulder, chest, and triceps

- Bodybuilding uses many techniques to increase the stress on your muscles, such as short rest periods and super sets. You should avoid these and allow yourself to recover well between sets. Normalise your heartbeat and avoid overstressing your body. **You will still get the benefits of increased insulin sensitivity** and muscle stimulation without harsher, more stressful measures.

- Allow ample recovery time. Do not exercise any muscle group more than once a fortnight at first, and never more than once a week, as this will have a counterproductive effect. Recovery is possibly the most important part of muscle building.

- If you feel a rise in symptoms or are exhausted, take a break for a week or two. Rebuild your walks before starting again with lower intensity.

One last thing: Get assistance and instruction, to make sure that you do your exercises correctly. Nothing is more annoying than a setback like an injury that won't even let you keep up your walking. But be careful about training with a personal trainer. The usual approach will not work for you, and they are not likely to understand the nature of CFS. My recommendation is only to use a trainer to ensure you are doing the exercises correctly, not to push you to work too hard.

Sports

Sports are dynamic, so controlling the intensity can be very difficult. Also, many sporting activities will take longer than my suggested maximum of 50 minutes.

If you are passionate about a sport, that is fantastic. Few things are better for you than having some fun. However, until you have made significant progress with your recovery, you have to be a little mindful to make sure that you don't overdo it. (Just don't be so mindful that you arouse your ANS.) In my experience, PECs are very excited to 'be back' and inevitably overdo it. I believe you are better off waiting until six to twelve months after full recovery before going back to sports.

Important notes for exercise recovery

Our focus on fat burning and muscle building is not for aesthetic purposes. You should not be concerned about body shaping or burning fat from your body. **What matters is the metabolic shift that will improve your health by reducing inflammation and increasing energy.**

Building up your fat-burning aerobic capacity will help you recover from CFS, but you will need to adjust your diet for it, since exercise and diet are intimately linked. Eating a balanced snack an hour before exercise is ideal to minimise the impact on your blood sugar. A snack after your workout, when insulin sensitivity is at its highest, is also a good idea.

Beware of your desire for carbohydrates. As you increase your activity, you will also increase your appetite. Whilst it is sensible to increase the complex carbohydrates in your diet, you must be careful to stay with complex carbohydrates and small, regular portions.

The timing of your exercise is also important. I believe that it's best to start exercising after 10 am and finish no later than 6 pm. If you start earlier, you run the risk of a low-sugar crisis and cortisol spike, as your reserves may still be low and your cortisol levels should be at their highest. Working out too late in the evening will stimulate your appetite, and the rise in cortisol could interrupt your sleep patterns. Sleep is one of the most important aspects of your recovery, so do not risk it by exercising too late in the evening.

It is critical to consider exercise for your recovery. The three biggest exercise mistakes that people make are as follows:

1. They do not exercise at all, which leaves them with an excessive glucose burden and a lack of detoxification, due to inadequate lymphasising.

2. They exercise too intensely, which directly triggers the fight-or-flight response in the overly-aroused ANS.

3. They exercise too much, which leaves them with depleted ATP reserves and too much oxidative stress. This leads to further mitochondrial dysfunction as well as exhaustion that indirectly triggers the ANS dysfunction.

Make exercise an important part of your recovery. Most importantly, have fun. Don't get too caught up in what you can or can't do, enjoy the activity, and look forward to doing more in the future at your own pace. It doesn't matter if you see progress within six weeks or six months. Exercise is only one aspect of your overall recovery.

Your health will not improve at a steady pace; instead, it will leap forward, then plateau, and even fall back a step or two at times. Enjoy the overall upwards trend and always, always listen to the messages your body sends you.

CHAPTER SUMMARY

- PECs can benefit from exercise to do the following:
  - Stimulate lymph fluid.
  - Reduce stress and lift mood.
  - Normalise blood glucose regulation and increase insulin sensitivity.
  - Rehabilitate the body.
- Stay within your energy envelope.
- Avoid metabolism pathways that break down muscles.
- Fat can be converted into glucose or burned directly. Burning fatty acids directly is more desirable. This occurs naturally at rest.
- Direct fatty-acid metabolism can be encouraged by conditioning the body via the following:
  - Making sure that enough carnitine is available.
  - Exercising at lower intensity (at a heart rate of around 60-65% of maximum).
  - Limiting carbohydrates, especially from grains.
  - Cutting out refined carbohydrates entirely.
- Yoga is an excellent exercise option for PECs.
- To minimise damage during aerobic training, always warm up for ten minutes to maximise fatty acid metabolism; then exercise for twenty minutes at 60% of max heart rate; and finally, cool down for ten minutes.
- Put off playing dynamic sports until your health is normal or near-normal.
- Listen to your body.
- If exercise increases symptoms, do less of it.
- Use weight training, but keep workouts short and focused.
- Exercise between 10 am and 6 pm.
- Focus on overall gains, not day-to-day progress and setbacks. Take a relaxed attitude and have fun.

CHAPTER 20

Lifestyle and Outlook are Everything

"Life... It tends to respond to our outlook, to shape itself to meet our expectations."

- Richard M. DeVos

The disruption in the functioning of the ANS is a result of too much stress. It's not just the types of physiological and psychological stress that we've mentioned, but also the stress of modern life.

Stress—like excessive exercise, bad food, and toxic exposure from our homes, the products we use, and the food we eat. Stress—like late nights, thanks to the wonder of electricity. Stress—like too much radiation from our homes, appliances, power lines, and mobile phones. No matter where we go, we see wireless communication and mobile phone towers.

Stress—like financial pressures to meet our complex and ever-increasing material needs. Stress from relationships that have been tested by chronic illness and financial pressures. Stress from our inability to live up to an image created not by ourselves but by a constant bombardment of media messages. Stress from worries about missing out, from the need to be constantly connected via phone, e-mail, Twitter, Facebook, and any other media we can get our hands on, often without forming real friendships and connections.

I have detailed many strategies to help you recover. The most important thing may be reducing the arousal of the ANS by addressing the stressors in your life and meditating daily. Other strategies, such as diet, supplementation, and exercise will help you leap ahead in your recovery.

However, your lifestyle and attitude are perhaps the most essential parts of your recovery. I have gone into so much detail to give you the information you need, but perhaps even more to give you confidence to approach this health challenge with a refreshed attitude and **the positive expectation that you will recover.**

Outlook for recovery

I know what it feels like to have CFS. I understand the worry and the fear that you will never overcome this 'mystery' illness. Whilst you have not recovered, you might think that something else is keeping you sick. Perhaps you have a bacterial infection that you need to get rid of, or perhaps your body is burdened by heavy metals. Maybe the expression of some gene has depressed an enzyme and you need to change your supplementation. And even if you can raise your methylation, how can you normalise the Krebs cycle without interfering with your cortisol production and thyroid function?...

PECs are not hypochondriacs, but we can sound like we are.

Many PECs know more than their doctors about specific aspects of physiology. But whilst much of your knowledge and efforts are correct, your focus on treatment and concern about the progress and problems with your recovery could do you more harm than good.

Your subconscious does not think in the same way as your conscious self. The subconscious is instinctual. You may understand intellectually that each thing is only a small part of the puzzle and that excessive stress cascades down to all the other problems and dysfunctions. But your subconscious sees only the focus on symptoms and health—a sign of danger.

You need to distract your subconscious by focussing your conscious mind on other things. If you have read this book and have confidence in its explanation of the cause of CFS, you will find it easier to move forward without undue concern, so that you can fully recover. But if you don't have confidence in it, then you may really struggle. That is why I have gone into so much detail to convince you.

Lifestyle adjustments: sleep

One of the most vital ingredients for recovery is good sleep. Sleep is critical to keep your mind and brain balanced, to replenish your hormonal glands, and to let your other bodily systems reset.

Lack of sleep alone may be enough to trigger CFS. I cannot overstate the importance of getting regular, restorative sleep.

Of course, it's not as easy as just going to bed early. The ANS dysfunction can cause cortisol surges late in the evening or in the middle of the night, which may wake you up and leave you unable to get back to sleep. Cellular dysfunctions can leave your body short of vital building blocks and adequate methylation to supply your brain with melatonin and to keep your other neurotransmitters in balance. Pain, discomfort, worry, and a racing mind can all keep you from the sleep you need to recover.

But you must do whatever you can to restore your sleep. Personally, I am against using medication for sleep, as I don't like the additional toxic burden or the poor quality of sleep it provides. You need deep sleep that leaves you feeling refreshed. However, if all else fails, you must explore all options, even if only temporarily.

In my personal experience, sleep improved as I recovered from CFS. It's a bit of a chicken-or-egg conundrum. However, a number of things can help you attract this powerful healing force:

- If you have not quit alcohol and stimulants, at least make sure that you do not have them after lunch. (I strongly suggest you quit them altogether during your recovery.)
- Have a protein-rich, low-carb snack around 8 pm.
- Create a good environment for sleep. Your room should have no light whatsoever, a good-quality, supportive mattress, a cool temperature, and no electronic entertainment of any sort.
- Don't drink more than occasional sips after 4 pm, and drink the majority of your fluids in the first half of the day. Make sure that you maintain adequate sodium levels.
- Establish a good bedtime routine.
- Aim to get into bed to sleep no later than 9:30 pm.

The makings of a good bedtime routine

The bedtime routine is an important step to help you sleep. Here are a few tips to help you:

- First and foremost, make it an actual routine, a ritual that is the same every night.
- Don't watch TV in the evening. It's stimulating, and the light from the screen will not signal your neurochemistry that it's time to sleep.
- Don't do anything too stimulating. Reading a novel is fine, but don't become creative or read nonfiction, as these will stimulate your mind.
- An hour before you go to bed, ideally around 8:00 or 8:30 pm, start winding down. Listen to relaxing music whilst brushing your teeth and getting ready for bed. Then, listen to a short guided relaxation and keep your mind clear as you ease into sleep.

If you really cannot sleep, don't stay in bed for hours. Instead sit, with a low-intensity, warm-coloured light and clear your mind by spilling your thoughts into a diary or onto a piece of paper; then perhaps read a little again before going back to bed.

Other options

You can encourage sleep by supplementing with 5-HTP or melatonin. However, you should only use these in safe amounts, and you must get medical advice before using them, perhaps even a second opinion. A better alternative may be the use of herbs, like valerian, lavender, lemon balm, chamomile, hops, or passionflower.

Other lifestyle adjustments

Search for balance in your life. It is easy to underestimate the impact of an unbalanced lifestyle. You must balance your work and private life, but also make sure that you have a social outlet, both with and without your family. It's also good to have a hobby. If you don't, try to reignite some previous non-sporting passion from earlier in life, or set a goal like learning a language or skill.

You might also like becoming closer to your community by getting involved in a charity or other project, but don't let this dominate your life. You may also find that pursuing your spiritual side will bring greater sense of balance.

Last but not least, you must have down time. I am not talking just about sleep, but about time at home doing nothing—not watching TV, not doing tasks, not cleaning, just pottering around the house or garden with no real agenda. Try it. It's very good for you.

Most importantly, be kind to yourself. Think of how you might treat a child after a traumatic experience or illness, and apply this to yourself. It's okay to have a break. Make sure you do something nice for yourself whenever you can.

CHAPTER SUMMARY

- Have a positive expectation that you will recover.

- Concentrate your efforts on treating the ANS dysfunction and don't get too caught up in other treatments.

- Getting regular, quality, restorative sleep is critical. To help you sleep, do the following:

  - Avoid alcohol and stimulants such as caffeine.

  - Have a quality, protein-rich, low-complex-carb snack around 8pm.

  - Limit fluid intake after 4 pm.

  - Create a good bedtime routine by avoiding evening TV, reading light fiction, meditating, or listening to relaxing music. Aim to get into bed to sleep no later than 9.30pm.

  - To encourage sleep, consider herbal remedies, melatonin, or 5-HTP, in small quantities under medical supervision.

- Focus on a balanced lifestyle that includes all aspects of life including work, family time, hobbies, exercise, learning new things, and rest and downtime. Also consider the spiritual aspects of your life.

CHAPTER 21

More Than One Way

"And I also trust that there's more than one way to do something."

- Dennis Muren

I f you have read the stories of people who have recovered from CFS, you will note that they have recovered in different ways. But if you look closely, you will see that they followed something akin to the guidelines in this book, even if they didn't realise it. Inevitably, they treated the central cause, the ANS dysfunction, by changing how they related to their illness and by reducing their primary stressors and triggers.

Let me share some stories of recovery with you to illustrate how different people have recovered. I compiled these from the experiences of many different people, with names changed to protect their privacy.

Mary's recovery

We met Mary earlier. Mary got progressively sicker and eventually stopped working. The stress of frustrated recovery and increased symptoms led to isolation and depression.

When the financial pressures got to be too much, Mary moved back in with her elderly mother. After six years of illness, she gave up on recovery. Her days were spent at home, avoiding anything that made her symptoms flare up and researching treatments on the Internet to help reduce her symptoms.

Mary became something of an authority on CFS and started a blog to give other PECs nutritional and supplement advice. After trying dozens of treatments over the years with varying success, she had fine-tuned her diet and supplementation. They kept her from being totally bedridden but they did not heal her CFS.

One Easter, her old friend Sandy asked her to join her at church. Mary explained that this was not a good idea, as it would likely make her feel worse. Sandy persisted, and after another heated argument with her mother, Mary decided to go, even though she was not very religious.

After the service, she met a small group of very nice people who asked her to join their Bible group. Mary explained that she wasn't comfortable with that sort of thing and found it difficult to get out as she was often unwell. Simon, the leader of the group, explained that they usually held the groups at members' homes and that they would be happy to meet next time at hers if she wanted. He said that Sandy thought Mary would help create some very interesting discussions.

Reluctantly, Mary agreed. Before she could call and cancel, they arrived at her place. To Mary's surprise, she really enjoyed the afternoon and considered meeting with the group again.

A month later, Mary had joined the group and really looked forward to the weekly meetings. One week, they discussed the power of faith for healing. Mary was deeply offended, given the extreme nature of her illness. Frankly, she didn't think her faith extended that far. The group united behind her and tried to convince her that there was a way to good health through God.

Mary was somewhat disgruntled, but she continued with the group. She also started going to church on Sundays and getting involved in other church activities. After three months, the group noted an improvement in her health and invited her to go on a church getaway. Mary had not been away from home for six years and, whilst very nervous, agreed to come along.

One evening at the camp, there was music and dancing. Mary ended up laughing and dancing with Simon for over an hour. When she went to bed that night, she felt great and realised she hadn't thought about her illness the whole weekend. She'd even forgotten to take her supplements that day. She wondered how she had managed to find all that energy and recognised that she hadn't had any symptoms the whole weekend. With her faith renewed, she prayed that night to thank God.

After that weekend, Mary had a relapse. But over the next few months, her health continued to improve. She eventually put it down to the power of faith. After six months, she started working part-time for the church. A little over a year later, Mary claimed she had recovered from CFS and was working full-time in a low-stress position that she enjoyed. That month she moved into a small apartment with the blessing of her mother.

Mary's renewed faith was important in her recovery. Her shift in focus and quiet time during prayer were instrumental. The supplements she was taking really helped spur her recovery once she reduced her ANS arousal.

Joan's recovery

Joan fell ill after her third pregnancy. It had been a difficult birth. At one point, they thought she would lose the baby. When she came home from hospital, Joan struggled to recover.

With her husband Andrew at work and three children under the age of three at home, she was busy, but her inability to recover baffled her. Over time, her condition got worse and she developed full-blown CFS symptoms.

Andrew tried to help her. They went from doctor to doctor without much result. In the end, she was diagnosed as having depression. On the advice of her doctor, her husband continually pushed her to get out and exercise in the fresh air, even though she felt she couldn't do it. Nobody seemed to understand the extent of her exhaustion. Her life was a constant stress between trying to cope with the children and feeling terrible all the time, not to mention the arguments she was starting to have with her husband. Both Joan and Andrew were worried that Joan might have contracted some sort of virus in the hospital that was causing her illness.

After several more doctors, Joan received a diagnosis of chronic fatigue syndrome. Nearly a year after that, she found Dr Olistico, who was different than the others. Her initial appointment lasted over an hour, as the doctor took a detailed history of her health. The doctor listened carefully and was very understanding. She explained that Joan's condition was not uncommon nor due to depression; it was due to extended postnatal fatigue. She was confident that Joan could regain her health with careful treatment, but explained that it could take up to six months. Joan and her husband were excited, although a little wary.

The doctor ordered many blood, saliva, and other tests, then prescribed a range of medicines for sleep restoration and pain relief, as well as a range of supplements. Joan was surprised by the number of pills and the cost, but on Andrew's insistence, she decided to give it a go.

During the third consultation, the doctor had a heart-to-heart talk with Joan and Andrew. As a result, Andrew cut back his work hours, and they hired a cleaner to help at home to give Joan some rest. They couldn't really afford it, but it would only be for a couple of months.

After about a month, Joan started to feel better. It was such a relief for both Joan and Andrew that they had finally found a doctor who knew how to treat her. The improvement gave Joan confidence that she had been correctly diagnosed and was on the right track. It was a weight off her shoulders. Their family life soon returned to normal, as Joan started to recover.

After only five months, Joan was back to her old self. She felt lucky to have found Dr Olistico.

Joan's recovery was due partly to the orthomolecular medicine that allowed her to rebuild her hormonal glands and support her mitochondrial function. Another part of it was due to the stress relief of getting help at home. All of this helped her to normalise her ANS dysfunction.

Michael's recovery

As a police officer, Michael was used to long hours and stress. But when he was transferred to an inner-city precinct, even he was shocked by the level of crime. He found it difficult to adjust, and his already-struggling marriage finally ended.

Shortly after the break-up, he and a female officer on patrol were overwhelmed by a gang. His partner was killed and he was badly beaten during the attack.

After being discharged from hospital, he still felt poorly, physically and emotionally, because he blamed himself for his partner's death. The department sent him to counselling, but it was the last thing Michael wanted.

Eventually he was well enough to return to work part-time in an administrative role. However, he felt he would never lose the stigma of what had happened.

Two years later, his health had really deteriorated. He went to doctors and had tests done, but they could find nothing wrong with him. That was strange, because he felt terrible and was in increasing pain. Eventually a specialist diagnosed him as having fibromyalgia. The specialist said that it might pass or might be a lifelong condition. Shocked, he went home and Googled fibromyalgia, only to feel even more dejected.

His condition got worse, but he stopped going to doctors, because they seemed to be of little help. About a year later, a friend who was a counsellor offered him TimeLine therapy sessions. She promised that he would not have to speak about the details of the day his partner died. Michael did not connect those events to his illness, but he finally agreed to address the trauma with her.

By his fourth appointment, he had started to feel much better about the terrible events. He had also enrolled in some pain management classes his counsellor had suggested to him and he was surprised at how these helped him to cope.

After one of his sessions, he walked into a health care shop. Susan, the shop assistant, was friendly (and attractive) and persuaded him to have a free naturopathic consultation with her. Michael had been reluctant to bother with this "voodoo" in the past, but now he didn't feel he had much to lose.

During the appointment, Susan did a live blood analysis and showed Michael that his blood cells were sticking together. She sold him some vitamin supplements, talked about the importance of diet, and invited him to a cooking class. Michael was glad to get out of the house and accepted the invitation.

Despite his reservations, he took the supplements for a short while and made some changes to his diet.

Five months later, Michael felt a weight had been lifted off his shoulders and he stopped seeing his therapist friend and going to the pain management classes. He had stopped taking the supplements as well, but he enjoyed his new diet and was feeling great. In fact, he became so passionate about cooking that when he was able to return to work, he resigned from the police force and started an apprenticeship as a chef.

Michael claimed his recovery was largely spontaneous. He didn't realise that not dealing with his trauma was suppressing his immune system and keeping him ill. Whilst he felt the pain management classes had helped him to cope, he didn't realise that the techniques were actually training his brain to sense pain normally again. The changes he'd made in his diet and in taking supplements also had had an impact on his biochemistry to support his recovery.

Becky's recovery

Becky had always been called "a highly-strung hippy". She had been the centre of social activity at university, but when her parents divorced, she put her studies on hold to travel to Nepal.

She was sick all through her holiday. Whether it was from the shots she'd had before the trip, the Nepalese food, or some sort of virus infection, she wasn't sure, but she had to come back early.

Becky never recovered, and her symptoms got worse, so she deferred another semester. She was living with her dad, who seemed increasingly impatient with her illness. Becky didn't believe in doctors but eventually, at his insistence, she went to see his general practitioner. The visit produced little result.

Weeks turned into months, until Becky had been sick for over a year. She refused to go back to the doctor. Instead, she went away on a meditation retreat with one of her friends, to get away from her dad. During that weekend, she was too tired to participate and slept most of the time. However, she met someone who told her about a fantastic detox program. He said he had felt exhausted for months, until he took the herbs and detox compounds prescribed on a certain website. He said they had detoxified his system and made him well.

Becky was completely convinced and very excited. She bought the products online and started the strict diet regime, although it meant having to give up her favourite Dr Peppers.

Within a month, Becky started to feel better. That gave her even more confidence that she was on the right track. After eight months of following the strict detoxing regime and other Eastern medical treatment, Becky had returned to full health.

Whilst Becky was convinced that her illness had been caused by a sort of toxic accumulation, her father's doctor dismissed this possibility.

Becky's diet and treatments did help her struggling liver, but the biggest changes occurred when she stopped having hypoglycaemic episodes. Her belief in the treatment was enough to reduce her concerns and symptom monitoring and to down-regulate her ANS dysfunction.

Frank's Recovery

Frank's story extends over nearly 25 years. He first got ill in his early thirties. His condition had stabilised since then, but he'd learned to settle for early retirement and living a limited lifestyle, to keep his symptoms to a minimum.

Whilst Frank described his health as reasonable, he had lost all sense of what it felt like to be normal. His life was limited mostly to weekly trips to the library and reading. He also went fishing with a friend once or twice a year, but those trips usually knocked him out for the next four weeks.

Then a friend sent Frank an e-mail about a centre specialising in CFS that claimed to be able to help people recover. Frank was sceptical. He'd long given up on treatments, having "tried them all", but the website had so many good video testimonials that Frank decided to give them a call.

The lady he spoke to was very friendly and said she would send him some information by e-mail. Unfortunately, the centre was halfway across the country. But Frank's cousin lived half an hour's drive away, so he decided to make an appointment.

Frank's wife Margaret came with him to his first appointment. However, Frank felt a little disappointed when the doctor explained what was involved and said that it would likely take some time for Frank to feel better.

The costs were significant, as they recommended he stay at the clinic for rest and a special diet as well as daily consultations. What worried Frank most was that the consultations sounded like some sort of group therapy. However, he met a couple of people who had received their treatment who were so positive and claimed such good results that Margaret eventually decided to sign him up.

Whilst reluctant, Frank invested in the program. The first two weeks were filled with more tests than he had ever had—blood tests, urine tests, hair tests, saliva tests, stool tests, and other ones he didn't even understand. He saw the clinic's doctor three times in the first fortnight.

Frank stayed with his cousin for some of the time to reduce the cost. His wife kept in contact by phone and visited once a month. After the third month of treatments, classes, and lots of doing nothing, Frank went home, but he stayed in touch with the centre to continue his treatment. He went back on three more visits that year.

Frank wasn't sure when exactly he recovered from CFS. Whilst he wasn't sure whether he had fully recovered or not, he was feeling better than he could remember. His wife noticed the biggest difference in him. Frank thought that his recovery was mainly due to the "pills and stuff", but Margaret felt that it was the overall program, including the group sessions where they did the "lifestyle education".

Many More Recovery Stories

If you wish to listen to people that have recovered from CFS tell their story in their own words, visit:

cfsunravelled.com

where many people have generously shared their intimate journey of recovery out of this illness, sometimes after decades of being ill.

CHAPTER 22

Summing Up and a Final Message

Having read all the information in this book, you might feel overwhelmed and ask yourself, "Now what?" So let me help you make sure that you got the main messages.

Look at your initial answers to the three questions:

1. What is the central cause of CFS?
2. What are the main things you need to do to recover from CFS?
3. Has doing these things led you to a full and permanent recovery?

I hope that the answers are clearer to you now.

I asked you to answer these questions before reading the book because it is easy, once we read and assimilate information, to convince ourselves that we already knew it. The problem is that if you already knew it, then it's nothing new and there is little for you to do.

You have to be clear about what you need to do to get better, and you have to take action.

The most important thing is to treat the ANS dysfunction, by identifying which of the listed causes apply to you and getting help from an appropriately-qualified person. Let me list them again:

1. Physical stress due to bodily dysfunctions (subconscious)
2. Mental and emotional stress about CFS and its symptoms (conscious and subconscious)

3. Mental and emotional stress from the environment (conscious and subconscious)

4. Mental and emotional stress experienced in the past (conscious and subconscious)

To remove the first cause (stress due to bodily dysfunction), diet, sleep, supplementation, and other medical and naturopathic support are critical. Whilst all dysfunctions and symptoms matter, few have as direct an impact as unstable blood sugar, so make sure you address this straight away. Remember, we are not talking about eating a strict diet forever, but just until you recover. After that, you can simply maintain a reasonable diet.

For the second cause (mental and emotional stress about CFS), it may be appropriate to see a psychologist, counsellor, or an NLP, TimeLine, or hypnosis therapist familiar with CFS. Practitioners all over the world specialise in treating this dysfunction; you just need to find them and make sure that their approach is on track. If a practitioner is not experienced with CFS, make sure that you focus your efforts on the real cause of the dysfunction, and not just on counselling to help you deal with having CFS. Learning to live with CFS is not the aim.

The aim is to stop triggering the ANS dysfunction and to recover. If you can't find specialised help near you, then you might consider investing in some self-help programs that teach you the skills you need to normalise this dysfunction. (You can find out more about the ANS REWIRE recovery program at the end of this book.)

For the third and fourth causes (present or past mental and stress), I recommend that you find help from a psychologist, counsellor, or NLP, TimeLine, or hypnosis therapist, depending on what the issue is. One of the greatest sources of stress is the experience of being unwell and its impact on the rest of your life, so this should decrease as you get better. But if you have other issues, please seek help.

You should also **learn meditation and practice it daily,** for at least an hour, as part of the normalisation of the ANS. It is unlikely that this alone will fix your problems, but it will certainly make the ANS normalisation a lot easier. **Without this practice, your recovery may be difficult.**

If you experience pain, learning psychological techniques to train your brain to feel pain normally can help. Pain is a major trigger.

Most PECs didn't get sick overnight, so you cannot expect to recover overnight. However, don't rule out a quick recovery, especially if you have been sick for less than a year.

Whilst you will always strive for better health, there comes a point when you have to let go of all this—a time when you have to stop talking to people about what is wrong with your health, and even to stop talking about what's right.

Many PECs do this instinctively, which is why I believe that you don't see so many stories of recovery on the internet. On some level, they realise that pretending it never happened is a better option than talking about it. Perhaps they fear that acknowledging that CFS exists, or that they used to have it, might bring it back. Perhaps they are right.

You can celebrate and appreciate your recovering health and lifestyle. You will naturally have a greater appreciation for health and the simple things in life—but take a balanced approach.

By "balanced", I mean that you can enjoy your health, but don't focus excessively on it. It must not be an obsession. At some point, you have to shut the door on your experience. Don't nudge the door or peek through the window at it; throw away the key and walk on. The connection between CFS and focus on your body and health is clear. Even when you focus on the renewed strength in your legs as you climb stairs, you are also scanning for signs of weakness.

And by "balanced", I mean you should remember the lessons you have learned to recover. Maintain a healthy, balanced lifestyle with joy, good diet, good exercise, and a positive outlook.

Good luck. I wish you a quick recovery and all the best that life can offer.

With love and best wishes,

Dan Neuffer

CHAPTER 23

CFS Unravelled: Questions and Answers

You should read this section only after you've read the rest of *CFS Unravelled* and understand its message about the root cause of the illness. Try to answer the questions in your own mind before reading the answers.

You may have further questions about CFS, but before you spend too much effort on them, consider whether having the answers is critical to getting well. Sometimes taking action is the most important thing.

Q: Why is my immune system depressed when nobody can identify a particular virus or other cause?

A: The immune system is initially depressed by too much cortisol. Whenever further cortisol surges occur, the immune system is further depressed, and over time, it can be damaged and function poorly. The deterioration of gut function and gut flora worsens the immune dysfunction.

Seventy to eighty percent of your immune system is in your gut, so gut dysfunction severely reduces the effectiveness of your immune system. Leaky gut, poor glutathione production, and opportunistic viral, bacterial, fungal, and parasitic infections all place further pressure on the immune system and leave it unable to cope.

PECs who fall ill following a pregnancy also experience immune system suppression as part of normal pregnancy. This may have contributed to your initial lower immune functioning.

Q: Why do I have a detox problem and have to eat nothing but green vegetables when that boozing, chain-smoking, pizza-gorging, binge-drinking party animal next door seems to be in perfect health, even following the worst of late-night benders?

A: Poor diet and toxic burden are not the only pressures on the detox systems of PECs. Others include too much stress, excessive cortisol, gut dysfunction, and other biochemical dysfunctions, such as mitochondrial and methylation problems. It is often more of a problem with our detox mechanism than just with toxic load.

Q: They tell me I have adrenal insufficiency. Why do I not get better when I treat it? Why, in some instances, do I actually feel worse afterwards? Why do other people who sleep less, work longer hours, and eat worse than I do, who are generally less healthy than I am, not have the same problem?

A: Adrenal insufficiency is not the problem; it is the body's interim solution to too much cortisol. Whilst low adrenal hormone output has negative impacts on your feeling of wellbeing, the real problem is the ANS dysfunction. You can treat the adrenal insufficiency and increase your adrenal capacity, but if you do this before you get rid of the ANS dysfunction, you may find that things get worse. You will simply have more cortisol available to flood your system.

Other people living a poor lifestyle may not get adrenal insufficiency for genetic reasons, but it's more likely due to low psychological stress or low levels of other physiological stressors. Your level of psychological stress largely depends on how you evaluate your environment and the meanings and rules you apply to situations.

Q: Why do other people seem to recover from CFS using a range of treatment and strategies such as the following;

- *Treatments for yeast infections or candida*

- *Treatments for irritable bowel syndrome*

- *Treatments for the adrenals*

- *Treatments to help detoxification*

- *Medication to restore sleep*

- *Medication to restore wakefulness*

- *Medication to make you feel happier*

- *Medication to kill viral infections*

- *Medications to kill bacterial infections*

- *Medications to kill parasites and infections*

- *Medications to reduce pain*

- *Vitamin supplements*

- *Mineral supplements*

- *Special diets*

- *Meditation and relaxation*

and why don't these work for me?

A: According to this hypothesis, the underlying cause of CFS is the ANS dysfunction. The real question, then, is not why some PECs don't recover using these treatments, but why some do.

I believe that these treatments reduce the dysfunction in some PECs' bodies enough to reduce their symptoms. This reduction in symptoms then reduces the physiological triggering of the ANS dysfunction. It also allows them to worry less and to reduce the focus on their symptoms to further help break the ANS dysfunction cycle. This is most likely because, first, they have faith in the treatment, and second, because they no longer have the mental or emotional stress that originally caused the ANS dysfunction. If no other stressors remain, any treatment that instils confidence and reduces symptoms enough could lead to recovery.

Q: *What is the central cause of CFS that cascades to cause all the other dysfunctions and symptoms?*

A: The ANS dysfunction is the central cause of CFS. However, long-time PECs may develop secondary problems, such as liver dysfunction, leaky gut, or mitochondrial dysfunction, which can help perpetuate the illness. These problems may also need to be addressed to achieve full recovery.

Q: *What are the main secondary dysfunctions that I must treat to overcome the central cause of CFS?*

A: Mineral imbalances, insulin resistance, hypoglycaemia, and mitochondrial and gut dysfunction are the keys to helping virtually all PECs correct the ANS dysfunction.

Q: *Why does my doctor not know about this, especially given that this all makes physiological sense?*

A: I suspect that it is for many reasons.

More and more doctors do understand CFS, but mainstream medicine is often decades behind medical science and is usually focused on reducing and treating symptoms rather than restoring health using the strategies outlined in this book. The modern model for doctor-patient interaction also makes it difficult for doctors to get involved on a deeper, more time-consuming way to help plan a complete recovery program.

Psychologists usually focus on helping people to cope with the symptoms rather than brain training designed to reduce them. There is great value in this and I have seen some people benefit wonderfully from such support. Cognitive behaviour therapy may be helpful in terms of reducing stress and coping with the illness. In order to change neuro-associations, beliefs, and habits, Hypnotherapy, NLP, and TimeLine therapy may be more effective. There are also other forms of psychotherapy that may be very helpful.

Therapists that understand the dynamics of CFS and the role ANS dysfunction plays, are in a great position to assist you with your recovery, especially if they have some intimate experience with the illness.

Another reason is that modern medicine judges the correctness and appropriateness of treatments based on a consensus of the majority, even if this does not offer the most value for patients. Support is growing for this explanation and for focussing on neuroplasticity as a path to recovery. You can encourage change by sharing this book and your experience of recovery with your doctor.

Q: What can I do to feel drastically better in less than 60 days?

A: This depends on what is happening with you individually. However, besides addressing the ANS dysfunction, taking significant amounts of quality magnesium supplements is likely to have the most dramatic effect, especially in PECs who have been ill for a long time. The next most obvious changes will likely occur by treating the gut dysfunction, by changing to a diet without dairy and wheat products for a time, taking probiotics to repopulate the gut, and eating more raw, low-sugar fruits and vegetables that contain enzymes. Normalising sodium levels where required may also have a dramatic impact in a relatively short period of time.

Q: If exercise helps, why do I feel worse when I exercise with any intensity?

A: During exercise, a body that produces too much or too little cortisol, has mitochondrial dysfunction, insulin resistance and poor blood sugar regulation, will quickly stop fatty acid metabolism. Instead, it will turn to glucose metabolism for energy, using anaerobic lactic acid fermentation, which causes excessive inflammation, blood sugar dysfunction, and more cortisol dysregulation. Whilst theoretically we may perform fatty acid metabolism at lower intensities (say, 60% of max heartbeat), most PECs are likely to switch out of this almost immediately. Changes in diet and exercise will help reduce this phenomenon, but you also need to address the ANS dysfunction.

Q: What are the key things that you must do while exercising if you are to recover from CFS?

A: You must stay within your energy envelope to maintain healthy ATP/ADP levels. Do not go into the glucose-burning mode that triggers inappropriate cortisol response. Also, you must avoid the severe energy shortfalls that reduce ADP to AMP.

Exercise in such a way that you always feel good when you finish. Do not do high-intensity exercise until your recovery is well underway. If you do weight training, proceed carefully, with short training sessions and good recovery between sets and training sessions.

Q: What further major health problems could arise down the road if you continue to live with CFS?

A: An acidic body, flooded by cortisol and under excessive oxidative stress, experiencing regular hypoglycaemic episodes, has an increased risk of a large number of "lifestyle diseases". However, if PECs correct these imbalances and adopt a healthy lifestyle which they maintain beyond recovery, I expect that they can achieve an above-average state of health.

Q: Can you be completely cured of CFS?

A: I don't think the word "cure" is appropriate. PECs can definitely regain a level of health that is average or better than average, which allows them to live a full and active life without CFS symptoms.

However, I believe that former PECs have the ability to recreate CFS more easily than people who have not had CFS. This is because PECs' bodies have created neural pathways and protective mechanisms of the nervous system which cause CFS. These are likely to remain available even if they are not active. In order to relapse, PECs would need to recreate the condition of excessive stress, most likely of multiple types. The important thing is to maintain a healthy, balanced lifestyle after recovery. **In my experience, people who understand why and how they recovered including the role of neuroplasticity, have a very robust recovery.**

Q: Do I have to settle for living with CFS as best I can?

A: Definitely not! I firmly believe that all correctly-diagnosed PECs can overcome CFS and regain a full and rewarding life, with the rich array of experiences life can offer.

My only caveat is that you may not be able to place yourself in unreasonably stressful conditions—such as living in a war zone, pursuing a high-stress occupation, or practicing an extreme-endurance sport such as running marathons—for extended periods of time.

Action Checklist

The second half of this book lays out a master plan for recovery. However, some people find this one-page checklist useful to jog their memory. My recommendation is that your first action be to reread this book.

ANS Normalisation	Medical/Orthomolecular Assistance	Diet	Exercise	Lifestyle
☐ Start daily meditation practice: • Take a course on meditation • Get meditation tapes ☐ Practice diverting attention from symptoms and stop body scanning. If necessary, seek help from: • NLP practitioner • Psychologist / counsellor ☐ Become mindful of unnecessary tension, including during physical tasks; learn to relax and belly-breathe. ☐ Start diary to identify emotional triggers. ☐ If you experience pain, get help from a pain psychologist to manage, cope with and normalise pain. ☐ If you suspect past emotional trauma, make appointment with: • Psychologist / counsellor • TimeLine therapist	☐ Find a holistic doctor or a doctor and naturopath who can work together. ☐ Review your medication and seek advice on its compatibility with supplements. ☐ Correct sodium/ potassium imbalances. ☐ Correct magnesium or other mineral nutrient deficiencies. ☐ Start a sustainable energy supplement protocol (including B vitamins and quality vitamin C).	☐ Eat three meals and three quality snacks a day. ☐ Eat balanced meals: 30–50% non-starchy vegetables and greens, and equal portions of proteins and carbs. ☐ Avoid sugary foods and drinks. ☐ Avoid caffeine. ☐ Avoid alcohol. ☐ Eat more non-starchy vegetables and low-sugar fruits. ☐ Eat fewer carbs, such as white potatoes, pasta, and rice. or eliminate them entirely. ☐ Eat more raw vegetables	☐ Make sure you exercise within your energy envelope. ☐ Listen to your body. ☐ Take a beginning yoga class. ☐ Take short outdoor walks. ☐ Once you are feeling better, have short weight-training sessions of medium-intensity only. ☐ Exercise between 10 am and 6 pm when possible.	☐ Eat a quality low-carb, protein snack around 8 pm. ☐ Drink the majority of your daily fluids before 4 pm. ☐ Start your bedtime routine around 8:30 pm. ☐ Avoid evening TV; replace it with fiction reading and relaxing music. ☐ Do some small thing each day that makes you happy. ☐ Find a hobby or passion that is exercise-appropriate. ☐ Make sure you maintain a balanced lifestyle as you regain your health.

List of Acronyms

This list is for your reference whilst reading this book. Please refer to it on an as-needed basis.

5-HTP   5-Hydroxytryptophan
           An amino acid that is the chemical precursor to serotonin

ACTH   Adrenocorticotropic hormone
           The hormone that stimulates the adrenal gland hormone release

ADP   Adenosine Diphosphate
           The reduced ATP molecule that gets recycled

AMP   Adenosine Monophosphate
           The reduced ADP molecule that can't be recycled

ANS   Autonomic Nervous System
           The part of the nervous system that acts subconsciously as the control system for the body

ATP   Adenosine Triphosphate
           The energy currency in the body

CFIDS   Chronic Fatigue and Immune Dysfunction Syndrome

CFS   Chronic Fatigue Syndrome
           The term used for ME, CFS, Fibromyalgia, POTS, CFIDS, and MCS

CNS   Central Nervous System
           The system in the body that consists mainly of the brain and the spinal cord

CRH   Corticotropin-releasing hormone
           The hormone that stimulates the pituitary's synthesis of ACTH

DHEA   5-Dehydroepiandrosterone
           A hormone released by the adrenal glands, gonads, and brain that is precursor to the sex hormones

EHS   Electromagnetic Hypersensitivity

GET   Graded Exercise Therapy
           Physical activity that starts very slowly and gradually increases over time; used by PECs

HPA axis   Hypothalamic Pituitary Adrenal axis
The mechanism that creates adrenal hormones

IBS   Irritable Bowel Syndrome

MCS   Multiple Chemical Sensitivity

NO/OONO   Nitric Oxide Peroxynitrate Cycle
The cycle postulated by Dr Martin Pall

PNS   Parasympathetic Nervous System
The part of the ANS that invokes the relaxation response

PEC(s)   Person(s) experiencing Chronic Fatigue Syndrome

SNS   Sympathetic Nervous System
The part of the ANS that invokes the 'fight or flight' response

About the ANS REWIRE Recovery Program

For years after I first published *CFS Unravelled*, I supported PECs by exchanging e-mails and by publishing recovery stories. Finally, I responded to calls for a recovery program rather than just ad hoc advice.

ANS REWIRE is my answer to that call. It is an online recovery program for ME/CFS, POTS, Fibromyalgia, MCS and EHS.

This education and training program is designed to help you get a deeper understanding of the dynamics of the illness so that you can partner more effectively with your health care professionals.

More importantly, the program trains you in specific techniques and strategies to effect the neuroplasticity required for ANS normalisation and a recovery of your health.

You can learn more about ANS REWIRE at:

ansrewire.com

where you can request to watch the four free introductory lessons of the program to help you take your first steps forward:

Lesson 1: Gaining Perspective

- Two internal challenges we need to overcome
- Three common bases for recovery that simply don't work and should NOT be pursued
- How an education/training program can be central to recovery from a severe physical illness

Lesson 2: The Explanation

- How the root dysfunction causes all the symptoms of ME/CFS/fibromyalgia
- How and why this driving dysfunction establishes itself

Lesson 3: Road To Recovery
- How the six groups of triggers perpetuate the syndrome
- The physical triggers that perpetuate the illness
- The scientific breakthrough that has only been accepted by the medical community in the last decades which paves the way to recovery

Lesson 4: Program Details
- The key requirement for change to produce recovery
- Three distinctions for recovery
- Content of and information about the ANS REWIRE recovery program

About the Author

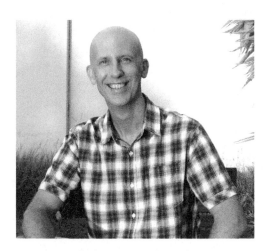

Dan Neuffer understands ME/CFS, POTS and Fibromyalgia intimately as he experienced the condition for 6½ - 7 years before recovering his health.

With a scientific background and training as a physicist, he dedicated himself to piecing together the 'mystery' of this syndrome which led to his ultimate recovery. Since his recovery he has dedicated his life to share his in-depth understanding and to use his unique insight from his own journey through the illness, to help others.

Besides *CFS Unravelled*, he also is the author of *Discover Hope*, and the cfsunravelled.com website. He has been conducting interviews with recoverers from all over the world to help inspire hope and direction for those experiencing the syndrome. His efforts to support others has culminated in the creation of the ANS REWIRE recovery program (ansrewire.com).

Dan lives on the Gold Coast in Queensland, Australia with his wife and two children. Having regained his life, he has a great passion for spending time outdoors with his family, fishing, hiking and family fun in the surf as well as engaging in those 'daddy projects' he could never do whilst he was sick.

Index

Did you love CFS Unravelled? Be the voice of change!

I wish I had known what I know now, when I was sick all those years. But finding the right information in a world of information overload can be tough.

If the explanation offered to you in CFS Unravelled really resonates with you, **please spread the word about the book to help others gain focus and hope for their recovery.**

There are 3 simple things you can do:

1.) Leave a comment on a ME/CFS/FMS/POTS website or Facebook page saying what you thought of the book (or write a review if you have your own website) with a link to cfsunravelled.com. This can have the biggest impact to reach more people.

2.) Ask your local library to stock the book. They usually have an online form that only takes a few moments to complete, or simply ask at the desk or on the phone.

3.) Write a review wherever you bought the book, or simply head to your local Amazon website and write a short review there.

Thank you for taking a moment to pay it forward to someone else who needs help.